U

Th

with Children

Using Story Telling

as a

Therapeutic Tool

with Children

MARGOT SUNDERLAND

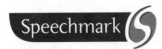

Speechmark Publishing Ltd
Telford Road • Bicester • Oxon OX26 4LQ • UK

Note on the Text

For the sake of clarity alone, throughout the text the child has been referred to as 'he' and the parent as 'she'.

Unless otherwise stated, for clarity alone, where 'mummy', 'mother' or 'mother figure' is used, this refers to either parent or other primary caretaker.

Confidentiality

Where appropriate, full permission has been granted by adults, or children and their parents to use clinical material. Other illustrations comprise synthesised and disguised examples to ensure anonymity.

Published by

Speechmark Publishing Ltd, Telford Road, Bicester, Oxon OX26 4LQ, United Kingdom
Tel: +44 (0) 1869 244 644   Fax: +44 (0) 1869 320 040
www.speechmark.net

© Margot Sunderland, 2000
Reprinted 2002, 2003, 2004, 2005

002–4720/Printed in the United Kingdom/1010

British Library Cataloguing in Publication Data

Sunderland, Margot
  Using story telling as a therapeutic tool with children.
  1. Story telling – Therapeutic use.   2. Child psychology
  I. Title
  618.9'8914

ISBN 0 86388 425 3
(Previously published by Winslow Press Ltd under ISBN 0 86388 274 9)

For Eleanore Armstrong-Perlman, whose remarkable empathy and understanding of troubled children has been a real inspiration behind this work.

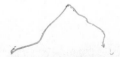

About the Author

Margot Sunderland is Founding Director of the Centre for Child Mental Health, London. She is also Head of the Children and Young People Section of The United Kingdom Association for Therapeutic Counselling. In addition, she formed the research project, 'Helping Where it Hurts' which offers free therapy and counselling to troubled children in several primary schools in North London. She is a registered Integrative Arts Psychotherapist and registered Child Therapeutic Counsellor, Supervisor and Trainer.

Margot is also Principal of The Institute for Arts in Therapy and Education – a fully accredited Higher Education College running a Diploma course in Child Therapy and Masters Degree courses in Arts Psychotherapy and Arts in Education and Therapy.

Margot is a published poet and author of two non- fiction books – one on *Dance* (Routledge Theatre Arts, New York and J Garnet Miller, England) and the other called *Draw on Your Emotions* (Speechmark, Bicester and Erickson, Italy).

Contents

Figures

Introduction

WHEN A CHILD'S too painful or too difficult feelings are left untalked about, they leak out in difficult and challenging behaviours, or in neurotic symptoms. Children do not have the inner resources to be able to fully process and digest their troubled feelings all by themselves. They need help.

To *process* painful and difficult feelings means to fully feel them and think about them, as opposed to avoiding feeling them, or giving them no real thinking time. If children are to process their feelings, they need an empathic adult who can offer them quality listening and understanding. In other words, they need an adult who makes every effort to *imagine in* to how the child is seeing things at any one time – an adult who takes the time to put themselves in the child's shoes.

Unfortunately, many adults have too little sense of how painful and difficult feelings need to be digested and worked through, just like food! So all too often children are left trying to cope alone. Their coping is so often a sad failure, causing much unnecessary suffering to themselves and/or the other people in their lives. This book – a vital resource for anyone working with children – is therefore about giving time to children's feelings through the vehicle of story. When a child is helped to think about his troubled feelings through story, it can prevent these feelings from building up into an awful mess inside. In other words, used well, stories can become a vital part of a child's healthy, *emotional* digestive system.

Chapter 1 addresses the philosophy and psychology underpinning the therapeutic value of story. Chapter 2 is all about practical ways of maximising the therapeutic value of telling a story to a child. Chapter 3 provides practical guidance on how to respond therapeutically when a child makes up a spontaneous story through his play. It is a chapter all about what to do and what to say.

As a note for people using this book who have no professional training in helping children work through their troubled feelings, I re-iterate the statement I made on this in *Draw on Your Emotions* (Sunderland, 1993):

A lot of excellent informal untrained counselling goes on in the pub, over the garden fence, or in the school playground. If the few people trained as therapists or counsellors were the only ones 'allowed' to listen to [children's] feelings, there would be far more suffering and loneliness in the world than there is today. However, having said this, some caution is vital. Emotional disclosure at any level must be treated with the utmost respect.

This is because, when children talk about their feelings, they are opening themselves up, letting down their defences and so becoming vulnerable. This means that any uninterested or low-key response; any faded response; any judgmental or critical response; any talking a child out of his feelings; any changing the subject; any taking over what he is doing or saying; can hurt a child. When a child has been hurt too much and too often by such responses, he will stop wanting to share his feelings. He may become very defensive and decide that any openness, or daring to be vulnerable is just stupid.

So, if you have no training in counselling or therapy, I strongly advise that you pay careful attention to the following sections in Chapter 3. They will act as guidelines for how to respond when a child tells you his feelings.

The sections are entitled:

- How to listen as a child speaks to you through story
- How to respond empathically to a child's story while staying within the metaphor

- The vocabulary to use in your empathic response
- The danger and damage of closed meanings

Although these sections are mainly focused on how to respond to a child telling you a story, they are also entirely applicable when a child is telling you his feelings.

So all that now remains for me to do is to wish you happy storytelling!

CHAPTER 1

The Therapeutic Value of Story

Why story is such a good way of helping children with their feelings

Being human inevitably means times of having some too difficult and too intense feelings. Some of these feelings can be so confusing, disturbing or painful that they are very hard to manage, let alone think clearly about, or work through. Yet, like food, such feelings need to be properly digested. If they are not, they can live on to haunt us in some way. They can spoil our relationships or interfere with our being able to function properly. They can bring too much unhappiness. This is because the energetic charge of these too difficult or too strong feelings does not just go away. Instead it gets bottled up inside, and as with all bottled up emotional energy, the problem is that it then leaks out in neurotic symptoms, body symptoms, or destructive behaviour.

This 'bottling up' then 'leaking out' can be even more extreme with children. Children do not have sophisticated coping strategies for dealing with their intense or too difficult feelings. They do not have the inner resources for thinking them through, or for regulating their levels of emotional arousal. We have endless examples of the painful consequences of this: bullying, aggressive behaviour, learning difficulties, bed-wetting, soiling, separation anxiety, problems with concentrating, uncontrollable behaviour, hyperactivity, obsessions, phobias, sleeping problems, nightmares, eating problems or a regular state of fear, anxiety or unhappiness. Any of these can develop unless children have help with managing and understanding their more troubling feelings.

So if children need help with their feelings, can't we just talk to them more about them? Herein lies the problem! Children do not talk naturally or easily about their troubling feelings, other than the odd 'Not fair!' or expressing anger with a furious 'No!', or by sulking, screaming or throwing something. Also, the few feeling words that children often choose, such as 'I'm bored', 'Cross', 'Fed up', or 'It's not fair,' tend to lead to a very restricted level of understanding from the adults to whom these words are being said. Very often these words misrepresent. Too often they are simply inaccurate. A child, for example, can spend years labelling his feelings with 'I'm bored', 'I'm cross,' mistaking these too limited reports for the truth, not realising that, as De Zulueta puts it so well, 'Experience lived is not the same as experience verbally represented' (1993, p131). Think also of the adult's frequent question to the troubled child, 'What's wrong?', and how the child often does not reply, *cannot reply*, in the language in which he is being asked to speak. Or he replies with a cursory 'Nothing's wrong' or 'I'm OK', which all too often shuts the door to help. Someone believes him, rather than thinking, 'Maybe he just hasn't the words to speak about how he is very much not OK.' Nor do young children talk to their little friends about their feelings.

The central argument in this book is that everyday language is not the natural language of feeling for children. Their natural language of feeling is that of image and metaphor, as in stories and dreams.

Toby, aged five

Mummy: 'Now, Toby, I want to try to explain to you about Daddy leaving.'
Toby: 'Look at that truck, Mummy!'

When she tries again later, Toby wants to show her the spider at the bottom of the toilet.

They are just talking in different languages – which the psychoanalyst Ferenczi (1931) calls a 'confusion of tongues'.

Sally, aged six

Sally is sitting in a café with her mother, who is talking ten-to-the-dozen to a friend about her anger towards her ex-husband. Sally is making circles in the sugar and getting her dolly to talk to the little pots of jam, which she is pretending are the homes of magic glow-worms. The adults are in the realm of thinking and feeling, and little Sally is in the realm of imagining and feeling. And so, when Mummy turns to Sally and says, 'Now look, Sally, we've got to talk about how you've been biting Sophie', Mummy gets nowhere. She is not speaking in Sally's language of feeling. Rather, she is using her own language.

Because of this language problem, many children fail to get the help they so desperately need with their emotional problems and troubled feelings. Furthermore, the adult trying to get through to a child with everyday language, regularly fails to reach the child in a way that shows that she *really* knows, or *really* understands. Rather, the child will tend to get distracted or feel lectured at.

So, if you want to speak to troubled children or have them speak to you, you are far more likely to be successful if you do it through 'their' language – the language of image, metaphor or story. Let us now look again at Sally and her mother:

Mummy: 'Now I want to explain to you why biting Sophie is wrong.'

Sally: 'Look at that little jam-pot, Mummy, it's got all yukky yuck on the side!'

Mummy: 'No, this is serious, Sally. Now listen to me [holds Sally's arm firmly], when you bite, it hurts . . .'

Sally: 'I'm having a big red balloon for my birthday, and one on my cake too!'

Mummy (persevering): 'So do you understand, Sally?'

> Sally says nothing, nods half-heartedly, but when Mummy lets her go, she continues in her fantasy world of magic glow-worm homes.
>
> Next day, Sally bites Sophie.

Sally's mother failed to connect with Sally in this interaction, for three important reasons:

- She is talking to Sally in the wrong language.
- She has not tried to understand why Sally bites Sophie.
- She has not given Sally another way of managing the feelings that made her bite Sophie in the first place.

This is where a story can get straight to the heart of the matter. It does so by addressing each of these three areas, as we shall see.

Using story recognises the limitations of talking about feelings to children in everyday language. Stories can speak to children on a deeper and far more immediate level than literal, everyday language. Talking about feelings in everyday language can mean going round and round in circles. This is because everyday language is a *language of thinking*, whereas speaking through a story, or playing out what you want to say with dolls or puppets, or through clay, a painting or in a sandbox scene, means you are *using a language of imagining*. This is the child's natural language.

For a child, everyday words and common feeling labels are often sensorially too dry. He is likely to experience them as dead little words. They are too flat, too reductionist, too cognitive to engage him. They are often also just not strong enough for the intensity of his, as yet undefended, way of being in the world. They fail to marry up with the sheer force of feeling he experiences from time to time. In the imaginative world in which he lives, which is so full of colour, magic, image, action, bright light and so on, dull little feeling words cannot hope to capture his emotionally charged, imaginative experiences. For a child, common feeling labels such as 'cross', 'sad' or 'scared' do little more than report feelings.

Furthermore, common feeling labels tend to 'flatten' what the child is experiencing into something which he is not. Think of trying to describe a beautiful daffodil in literal words, for example. This makes it far less of a daffodil. It is stripped of its essence; its sensuality; its complexities, and the directness with which it affects us:

> The soul wants imaginative responses that move it, delight it, deepen it. (Hillman, 1983, p38)

> The earth is not flat and neither is reality. Reality is continuous, multiple, simultaneous, complex, abundant and partly invisible. The imagination alone can fathom this and it reveals its fathomings. (Winterson, 1995, p151)

In contrast, stories told by adults to children, or children telling stories to adults through play or painting, can speak about feelings with amazing richness. In fact, the mind naturally speaks about emotional issues through story, as we see in dreams. In dreams, image and metaphor are the mind's *chosen* way of processing powerful feelings in our past or present, as well as our fears or hopes for the future. A story is simply like having a dream while being awake.

Take, for example, Tessa (aged 5), who regularly has major temper tantrums on the floor in the supermarket. Afterwards, Tessa is in a very frightened state because of the intensity of feeling inside her. She often has nightmares about monsters that same night. The adult response of 'You seem very cross' says far too little about *what* and *how* Tessa is actually feeling. It fails to convey the full *qualitative and energetic* aspects of her tantrum experience. The word 'cross' is too vague, too generalised. It is a dead word. As Hillman says, it is 'a terrible impoverishment of the actual experience' (Hillman, 1983, p44). But tell 'temper-tantruming' Tessa a story about floods or avalanches, or a fire that rips through everything, and you will probably find you get through to her and convey to her that you understand something of what she has been going through. Or ask Tessa to tell you a story, paint a picture or make something in clay, and you are asking her to speak about her vitally lived experience.

In fact, as well as children, many adults get stuck in the cul-de-sacs of convenient feeling labels to describe their *own* feelings. Toned-down feeling words, or very oblique or minimising references to intense emotional states or experiences, are also arguably part of our repressed culture as a whole, as expressed here in part of a poem by Jacqueline Brown:

> Even words were counterfeit – 'a visit from your
> Auntie', 'a number two', 'hanky-panky' and 'passed
> away' were cheap plastic versions of blood, shit,
> sex and death that might shatter and cut.
> We were force-fed the fake for so long it was hard
> to recognise the real when we finally met it
> ('Imitation', 1996, p46)

In short, parent-child, teacher-child or counsellor-child communications about feelings when only everyday language is used, are likely to be impoverished. The conversation will tend to lack depth of expression and understanding on both sides. It will have none of the subtleties, the complexities about felt life from a communication spoken in the realm of the imagination. If literal words were completely adequate in expressing what we human beings feel, there would be no need for art or music or theatre or poetry. But of course they are not. The following are examples of cases where everyday language failed to reach a troubled child, and where story got through.

Charlie, aged six

When Charlie was five, his father moved out to live with his new partner abroad. It was a sudden parting, because the marriage was in an awful state and Charlie's parents thought it would be damaging to Charlie if they were to stay together any longer. Charlie loved his Daddy intensely. But when his Daddy moved out, Charlie just got on with his life. He did not cry, and seemed to refer to his father only in a matter-of-fact way. However, his school work deteriorated dramatically, and teachers often found him just staring out of the window. His mother and other relatives tried endlessly to get Charlie to talk about Daddy leaving. They failed. When they said to Charlie how they could imagine how sad and cross he was, Charlie just got on with polishing his bike, or playing with his Ninja Turtles. These adults' words seemed to have very little impact on Charlie.

The problem was, Charlie's mother and her relatives were using the wrong language. They did not realise that Charlie needed to deal with his feelings through image, story and metaphor, and was in fact already doing so:

- Most nights Charlie dreamt of being with Daddy, and then suddenly along came a giant sheep and kidnapped Daddy. In other dream scenarios Daddy would die in a car crash on his way to see Charlie.
- Most days, Charlie said to his mother, 'Can we have that story again tonight? The one about the little bear that gets stuck in the black hole until everything turns awful, and he can't see the sun any more?'
- Most days, Charlie asked, 'Can we watch the film *Titanic* again?'. And when there was no time to watch *Titanic* again, or his mother said 'No', as she was getting sick of watching it, Charlie said, 'Well, can we just watch that bit when the couple lose hands with each other and get separated?'

In short, Charlie's mind was saying, 'Look, I need to deal with this trauma, but I need to deal with it through image, metaphor and story'. (A dream, of course, is also a made-up story.) It was via story that Charlie was busy processing his feelings about his Daddy leaving. His mother's attempts at connection were sincere and genuine, such as 'I think you are probably very sad about Daddy moving out', but they simply labelled Charlie's feelings. Her words failed to speak about the fuller, deeper picture of what Charlie was feeling. Unlike the images in the stories Charlie chose to keep revisiting, his mother's words neither touched nor moved him. He was left feeling she did not understand the depth of his pain.

Eventually, with the help of a professional counsellor, Charlie's mother got the idea about Charlie's chosen language of story, image and metaphor. So they watched the fateful scene in *Titanic* together, but in a different way this time; his mother now appreciating its symbolic significance for her son. When they talked together about it,

Charlie wept and wept. 'He just wanted to hold on,' he cried. 'He just wanted to hold on! Why did he have to let go? He could have kept joined up if he had really, really wanted to.'

Charlie and his Mummy both knew that he was using the tragic couple in the film to talk about him and his Daddy. But his Mummy had the sensitivity to let him stay within the metaphor for as long as Charlie needed. After she had gained his trust this way, by waiting and just being there, he cried, 'I miss my Daddy so much. How dare he leave me!'

Gemma, aged four

Gemma: 'Mummy, I'm frightened of monsters getting me in the night.'
Mummy: 'Gemma, there aren't any monsters. Believe me, darling.'
Gemma: 'Yes there are!'

After this conversation, that night Gemma was again terrified of monsters eating her up when she was asleep – just as she has been many nights before.

Gemma's mother had not managed to connect with Gemma for a number of reasons:

- Her mother is mistaken: there may be 'no monsters' in Gemma's outer world, but there are in her inner world!
- Her mother has not tried to understand what in Gemma's outer or inner life is making her so frightened of monsters. Is she being bullied (outer life)? Or is she frightened of something she perceives about a relative or teacher? Or is it her own monsters she fears (inner life) – in the sense that children can often fear the strength of their own passionately angry feelings?
- Her mother is talking to Gemma in the wrong language.
- Her mother has not given Gemma an alternative way of speaking about or coping with her feelings about monsters.

Gemma needs help in tackling her monsters, but *in the realm in which she is experiencing them – the realm of her imagination*.

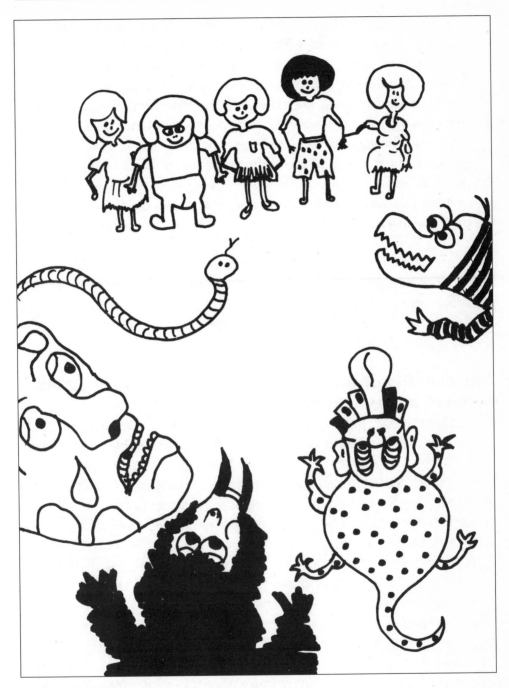

Figure 1 *When monsters are easy-peasy*

With the help of a friend, Gemma's Mummy found a book called *I'm Coming to Get You*, by Tony Ross, an excellent book about monsters. This is a story about literally reducing 'monsters' to manageable size. After hearing the story, Gemma got out some of her toys and enacted a story about monsters. She called it 'When Monsters are Easy-peasy' (see Figure 1). She told how she and an army of friends defeated the monsters. Through her story, she was rehearsing feeling powerful and supported in the face of awful threat, rather than alone. Her fears subsided, and it was all done in the realm of the imagination.

It is a powerful combination: a story told to the child, and then the child enacting a story back, which is in fact her own inner story.

'It is my belief that all presenting problems and symptoms are really metaphors that contain a story about what the problem really is. It is therefore to create metaphors that contain a story that contains the (possible) solutions. The metaphor is the message' (Heller & Steele, 1986, quoted in Mills & Crowley, 1986, p50).

The benefits of telling therapeutic stories to troubled children and why they work

A therapeutic story can work as an 'admission ticket' into a child's inner world. The ticket is often granted, in the sense that, with a well-chosen story, a child will listen intently because you are entering his feeling world with care and understanding. Telling him a story can feel far more respectful and far less invasive than a statement such as, 'Now let's talk about how sad you are that Daddy has left home', or 'How do you feel about your Daddy divorcing your Mummy?'

A therapeutic story speaks of common emotional issues and problems, but it speaks of these within the realm of the imagination rather than within the realm of cognition.

A therapeutic story aims to speak with empathy and precision about the emotional issue or problem with which a child is struggling. Unlike everyday language, it speaks through highly charged expressive images. In so doing it can capture the fuller picture, the deeper realities of a child's emotional experience. It can capture the multisensory and essential energetic qualities of a feeling or emotional event: its atmosphere, tensions, tones, intensities, ebbs and flows, crescendos and diminuendos, urgencies and dynamic shifts. In the words of the poet Seamus Heaney, a therapeutic story can therefore 'amplify the music of what happens'. Everyday language and common feeling labels often miss whatever is of central importance to a child in the painful or difficult experience he is going through, or they only make passing reference to it. In contrast, the therapeutic story is often a profound form of description and evocation of the child's inner world of image and feeling.

A therapeutic story can therefore enable a child to see, hear, know and feel more clearly, by providing a deeper truth and empathy than is possible through literal words. In so doing, it can bring hope to a child that 'I can be understood. It is worth telling someone about my feelings. At last I've got through!'.

> I believe that art puts down its roots into the deepest hiding places of our nature and that its action is akin to the action of certain delving plants, comfrey for instance, whose roots can penetrate far into the subsoil and unlock nutrients that would otherwise lie out of reach of shallower bedded plants. (Winterson, 1995, p35)

A therapeutic story speaks to a child about how a coping mechanism he is using is costing him too much. For example:

- Bottling up his too troubled feelings
- Exploding
- Giving up, not caring
- Becoming hard and tough so as not to feel pain any more
- Just allowing himself to be bullied or abused and not telling anyone
- Giving his life over to something or someone who is causing him too much hurt

Yet it is perfectly understandable that a child uses one or more of these coping mechanisms, as he does not have the inner resources to cope in a healthier or more creative way. Hence the need for the therapeutic story. A therapeutic story speaks to a child about how a coping mechanism he is using is making him very stuck. A therapeutic story also speaks to a child about how his coping mechanism has brought him to a point of crisis. (This is shown by the main character in a story coming to a crisis point because of his coping mechanism, as in Figure 2.)

Yet the hope for the listening child is that the main character in a therapeutic story does persevere after reaching rock-bottom. The message is strong and clear: *don't give up*. There is always something 'around the corner' to help you, which, because it is just around the corner, you cannot quite see right now.

A therapeutic story presents hope and possibility in the form of healthier, more creative coping mechanisms and ways of being. In so doing, a therapeutic story can transport a child into a fantastical world, a magical world. But it is a world that contains more than meets the eye. The psychological processes represented by the characters and their adventures in these worlds are packed with meaning. If a child is open to it, he can enter through the story world into a world of hope, of options and of possibility. In the story world he can find tools for a richer and more satisfying future. He may choose to leave these 'tools' lying there, or he may pick them up and start to use them in his life, now or at another time. This is how a successful therapeutic story will work for a child on an inner level:

- It presents options about what to do when you face a huge obstacle in your life.
- It presents new possibilities, creative solutions for tackling and overcoming seemingly insurmountable problems.
- It shows ways of dealing more effectively and far less painfully with very common emotional problems.
- It provides options for new ways of being.

These new ways forward may not be acted on in the child's life right at that moment, but can act as a seed planted in his mind, taken in as a resource, and lived and used fully in later life.

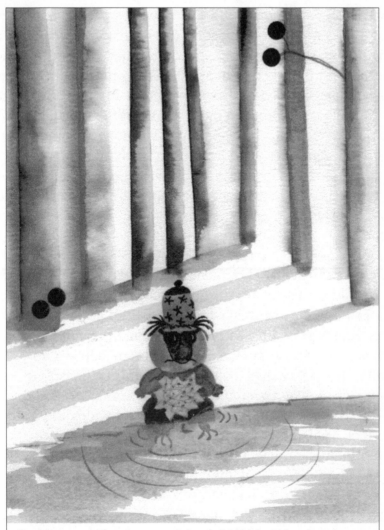

So Bipley sat by the grey lake in Wibble Wood and thought and thought. 'If I keep the tough stuff around my heart, I need never feel hurt again. But then having the tough stuff around my heart means that I can't feel any of the beautiful things in the world.' Bipley was very, very stuck. It felt like he was sitting next to the biggest problem of his life.

Figure 2 *Bipley's crisis*

A therapeutic story offers a child new ways of thinking about his troubled feelings. The story presents these feelings which have already been rigorously thought about, by the author. This is by and large extremely useful to the child, who is likely to have had these troubled feelings without being able to think them through. So therapeutic stories can allow children to move into a different way of seeing a situation, of knowing it, or of relating to someone or something in their lives. Stories therefore provide a child with time to reflect on his situation, his feelings and ways of being. Every painful or too intense feeling needs time for reflection. A therapeutic story provides that time, whereas, if an adult tries to give straight advice to a troubled child about the way to deal with his feelings, the child may not be able to hear, or may ignore, avoid or in some way spit it out. A therapeutic story therefore offers knowing about feeling and emotional literacy in a way that is usually made far more palatable to the child by creating vivid pictures in his mind, enabling him to identify with the story's main character who is grappling with the very same difficult feelings as he.

A therapeutic story can enable a child to dare to stay with the disturbing, the too intense, or the too painful feelings *long enough to really think about what is happening,* when his first inclination is to run away. This is because metaphorical image provides the means for a child to look at his powerful feelings from a 'safe distance'.

A therapeutic story includes very important psychological messages. In this sense, a therapeutic story is allegorical. Aesop's *Fables* were allegorical, but often also harsh and judgmental: for example, 'You're bad if you do this, and good if you do that.' A therapeutic story, however, is designed primarily to empathise with the child, not to blame or wag the finger. It presents important psychological messages concerning a common dilemma, problem or existential crisis in the life of a child. For example:

- How to be open to love and yet still be able to defend yourself against people who want to hurt you.
- How to love, in terms of bringing you more happiness than pain; who to love, and how to break an addiction to someone who cannot love you.

- How you can change your fundamental way of being in the world.
- When to let things be and let things go, and when to challenge and confront.
- How much to go after what you really want in life, and how much to just stick with the status quo.

A therapeutic story also often has important psychological messages about permissions. For example:

- You have every right to say 'No', or 'I do mind'.
- You can be different.
- You can follow your dream, even if people say to you that it is far too wild and that you will never make it.
- You can change the way you feel.
- You can be free of anxiety.
- You can let go.

Using a therapeutic story also models a calling on imagination to help with too difficult feelings. The imagination often has far more useful things to say about feeling than has cognition. In times of emotional stress, mental rumination simply tends to churn out the same old answers, anxieties, self-put-downs, and critical inner voices.

A therapeutic story can speak about a child's 'unthought known' (Bollas, 1987). The unthought known is a sense that, 'I know this exactly, but I have not ever thought it.' It is when you look at a painting; hear a piece of music; see a film; witness an emotional event, and feel 'Wow, it's speaking about something I know deeply.' It touches you profoundly, yet, try as you may, you are unable to find the memory that is causing the resonance. When a child gets this from a story, the story gives him a sense of being profoundly understood. It is a sense of real relief. When an 'unthought known' can be named, then it can be thought through and felt through.

Tommy's teacher read *Willy and the Wobbly House* (Sunderland & Armstrong, 2000) to Tommy. It is a book about a very anxious little boy who finds a very calm Puddle Queen who takes Willy in her arms and soothes him. After the story Tommy said to his teacher: 'You know what! I feel like Willy sometimes, I mean all jelly-wobble inside, especially when my Mummy goes away for a long time. But I never knew it was a jelly-wobble feeling before. It's not so scary, now I know. And maybe I'll just ask Mummy for an extra-long cuddle before she goes away for a long time, so that she can be my Puddle Queen in my mind, while she's not there.'

So in Tommy's case the story brought his 'unthought known', highly anxious feelings into a conscious awareness of his anxiety that could then be properly processed. An 'Aha!' insight born out of creative imagination in this way, instead of being born out of dry thought, is far more likely to be a felt and long-lasting realisation.

As Moore says, 'The soul of a piece of art is known intimately, not remotely. It is felt, not just understood' (1992, p291). The same is true of stories! In summary, children desperately need emotional education, and until this is formalised in some way on all school curricula, it is to be hoped that the therapeutic story can go some way towards offering such education.

How does a child actually listen to a therapeutic story?

How does the empathy get through, and how do the learning and the healing happen? First and foremost, if a therapeutic story is aptly chosen for a particular child, he will identify with the main character in the story. In so doing, he will go on the same journey as the character. He will suffer that character's defeats and obstacles, but also feel the character's courage to continue. As the child goes along the journey with the character in the story, he no longer feels alone with his problems and his too painful or too difficult feelings because, hey presto! the character in the book is having them too. This character is getting into a horrid stuck place because of the way he is dealing with the problem, just as the child feels he is getting into a horrid stuck place with it too. But eventually the child will feel the character's joys and relief in coming through conflict and crisis to a place of resolution.

Sarah is a little girl, aged six, who misses her Daddy terribly

Sarah's Daddy walked out one day to go and live with another woman. He did not contact Sarah. He did not reply to any of her letters. She yearned and longed for a response. Sarah's Aunty read to her *The Frog Who Longed for the Moon to Smile* (Sunderland & Armstrong, 2000). It is about a frog who is in love with the moon because once the moon smiled at him. Now he spends all his time gazing at the moon in the hope that the moon will smile at him again. You can imagine how easy it was for Sarah to identify with Frog in the story; how, on hearing the story, she found that it was charged with meaning for her. Sarah knew Frog's feelings only too well, so her identification with Frog was very deep. In the book, with help, Frog moves through to a new place. The story opens up, offering a new, more hopeful picture of a previously very painful situation. By identifying with Frog, Sarah was enabled both to grieve for her Daddy and vicariously to explore different ways of being with her painful feelings. She started to think and feel about different ways of responding, and so moved out of her stuck position regarding her relationship with her father.

After hearing a carefully chosen therapeutic story, the child now has two pictures of his painful situation in his head: the old picture – pre-story – and the new picture – post-story – enriched by all the empathy and creative possibility the story has provided. Sometimes, in the child's mind, the new picture can blend with the old, and sometimes the new can eclipse the old. But certainly, when the story has really caught the child's attention, he has the images of a new hope in his head as well as his old hopelessness, confusion, 'stuckness', or overwhelming pain. In this sense, a good therapeutic story can be a real emotional support to a child. You know this is happening when the child says 'Read it again and again and again.'

The messages get through because a therapeutic story uses indirect expression – and herein lies its power:

The fatherless child crying through the farewell scene of *E.T.* may never consciously think, 'This is just like when Daddy went away.' Yet on some level the sense of love and ultimate well-being suggested by the movie's ending may help the child to experience his loss in a new and more healing way – and without his ever being aware of it. (Mills & Crowley, 1986, p65)

The indirect expression of a therapeutic story is where both its safety and its wisdom lie. To explain, using a story to help children with their feelings is like saying, 'Let's look at these characters' lives, rather than directly at you.' This way the child does not feel exposed in the spotlight, embarrassed, humiliated, got at or shamed. After all, it is the character in the book that is feeling X or Y, isn't it? The most successful stories are the ones that are absolutely right in terms of speaking about the pain with which the child is busy grappling, both on a conscious and an unconscious level (the latter being evident in his dreams, or in his acting-out behaviour his neurotic symptoms).

The paradox of indirect expression directed straight at the child, means that a story can affect him on both these levels: consciously and unconsciously. And it is often on the latter level that he receives the therapeutic message from the story. 'In the Persian language there is a saying that can be translated as, "One tells something to the door so that the wall will hear it"' (RowshaM, 1997, p50).

Imagine telling a story to a little girl, aged four, about her bed-wetting problem, but a story with no indirectness via metaphor, images and characters: 'There was a little girl with a bed-wetting problem. Every single night she wet the bed.' Frankly, this is an attack on the child's dignity. It also has none of the power of indirect expression, the power of metaphor. It just *reports* the child's situation; it does not symbolise it. Also it is as if you, as storyteller, are giving the message, 'I'm OK because *I* don't wet the bed and *you're not* OK, because you do.' A therapeutic story has absolutely none of this judgmental flavour.

In short, a literal story about bed-wetting will not help the little girl, and may well cause damaging shame or humiliation. However, a story about the feelings of wetting the bed taken into an imagining realm, away from its habitual context, allows the little girl her privacy and dignity, coupled with the fact that solutions can be embedded in the story with subtlety and ease.

I made a mistake once in telling a story to a little girl who had gone through awful traumas in her life. I told her a story to convey my empathy about the terrible fear and aloneness she had experienced. I translated into metaphor – that is, into indirect expression – things like the abuse from her father, and the cruelty of her mother who would make her sleep on bare bedsprings when she wet the bed. (In the story, I used images such as hawks who swooped down and put sharp screeching noises into the ears of a child and took away her teddy. I spoke of cruel skunks who robbed the child of all that comforted her.) The little girl was completely engrossed. Right at the end, I named the child in the story with the little girl's name. She rushed out of the room. I had blown her cover, and taken her into the realm of shame and exposure. It was a vivid lesson for me about the need for indirect expression.

Chapter 2

How to Use Storytelling as a Therapeutic Tool with Children

How and when to tell a therapeutic story to a child

Tell a therapeutic story to a child when you have his full attention, when he is open and receptive to it, not distracted by wanting to do something else or be somewhere else. At bedtime, if you have a story time, do not worry about disturbing a child with a therapeutic story before he goes to sleep. Remember the therapeutic story is an indirect expression, and children often feel relieved after hearing one, because of the built-in empathy and resolution at the end.

In a school, it can be good to have a special place in the room just for stories, so the child quickly associates this place with calm, and with story. Point to the action and characters in the picture as you read, so that the child can follow what is happening visually.

Be sensitive to occasions when a child may want to linger with a picture or part of the story. This often happens with therapeutic stories, so avoid turning the page until you feel the child is ready. Some therapeutic symbols may speak very loudly to a child, so let him take these in. If a child wants repeated telling of the story, that is a very good sign: it means he is really thinking and feeling about its message; he is making it his own, imbuing it with meaning from his own life and circumstances. Bettelheim writes that only after repeatedly hearing a story, 'will the child's free associations to the story yield the tale's most personal meaning to him, and thus help him cope with problems that oppress him' (Bettelheim, 1975, p58).

After you have read the story, do not come out of the metaphor, unless the child does. Do not say 'Frog is like you, isn't he, because you miss your Mummy like that, don't you?' The child may feel shamed and exposed if you do. Also he can identify with Frog perfectly well on his own. Remember that the 'indirect expression' of a therapeutic story is usually where its power lies. It is fine, of course, if the child brings it out of the metaphor of his own accord, and says something like, *'I feel a bit like Frog sometimes, when I'm missing Mummy.'* Then he is giving you licence to talk with him about this directly, rather than indirectly.

I am often asked, 'But *can* a child change, if I always stay in the metaphor, and if I never ask him, "Do you ever feel like the character in the book?"' The answer is yes. I have seen it happen many times. The story's meaning is working away in the child's mind on a subconscious level, just as dreams at night are metaphorical stories in which a child is working through important emotional experiences. If the story has resonance for a child, and he is in an open, receptive state while it is being read to him, the story will indeed have an impact on him – an impact that can keep working in his mind long after the story has finished.

How to think up your own therapeutic story for a child: A simple guide to constructing a therapeutic story

Not all therapeutic stories follow this construction, but it is a very common and workable one. First, identify the emotional problem or issue with which the child is grappling (see the list on pp23–24). Now think of characters, a place, and a situation that can provide a metaphorical context for this problem or issue. Then present the main character as grappling with the same emotional problem or issue as the child.

Show the main character using coping strategies for the problem or issue similar to those coping mechanisms used by the child. Show how these coping mechanisms lead him into troubled waters or down the wrong road or cul-de-sac, which is self-destructive and/or destructive to others. Show the ultimate failure of that coping mechanism which results in the character reaching some kind of internal or external crisis in his life. (The story so far should have captured the whole context of how that character *came* to that moment of crisis in his life.)

Show the journey from the crisis to the solution of the crisis. Beware of moving too quickly from problem to solution – in other words using 'quick fixes'. There must be a journey, a bridge between the two. Without this, the story becomes unbelievable and not like real life at all.

Next comes the shift: usually as a vital part of the journey towards solution, someone or something appears in the story that helps the character to change direction and move on to a better coping mechanism, or a far more creative way of dealing with the situation. The main character then successfully adopts a new behaviour, way of being or coping mechanism, and feels a lot better. It alters his experience of himself and of others. The world is a far better place to be.

How to identify and choose the correct emotional theme for your story

For a therapeutic story to have a deep psychological impact on the child, it must speak to him about the emotional issues he is busy grappling with, and also about his current ways of coping, which are costing him too much. So, ideally, before you tailor-make a therapeutic story for a child, know the emotional themes that come up again and again in his play; know the emotional themes in his dreams; his neurotic symptoms, or acting out behaviour.

Below is a list of very common emotional themes that trouble children. Pick the one(s) that your child is grappling with and this will become the emotional theme of your story:

- Feeling not wanted
- Feeling powerless or insignificant
- Feeling 'unspecial', unimportant or invisible
- Feelings of being the unfavoured one
- Feelings of not belonging

- Feeling not liked, or actively hated
- Feeling rubbished, abused, used
- Feelings of self-loathing
- Desperately wanting someone to like me or love me who doesn't
- Feelings of needing someone too much
- Feeling lonely
- Feeling broken-hearted
- Feeling emotionally hungry
- Feeling lost
- Feeling empty inside
- Always needing to be in control
- Always anxious about something
- Feelings of fear about anything new or different
- Worrying that Mummy or Daddy might die or leave me
- Trying to 'mend' Mummy and Daddy because they are ill/depressed
- Feeling 'I want to run away or hide'
- Living in fear of doing something wrong
- Living in fear of doing something shameful or embarrassing
- Feeling trapped
- Feelings of wanting walls to keep others out
- Living in fear of being bullied/bullied again
- Feeling that the world is basically a frightening place
- Feeling that no one or nothing is safe
- Feeling invaded or taken over
- Feeling contaminated
- Feeling uptight, angry or that I am sitting on a volcano
- Feelings of wanting to hit out, hurt or destroy
- Feeling that 'It's all too much'
- Feeling that I am trying to hold up the world
- Feeling a mess inside
- Feeling that 'I am bad'
- Fear of being myself in case I damage someone
- Feeling 'What is the point of anything?'

More on how to use indirect expression in your story

Next, in order to transform the literal into the symbolic, take the emotional theme or issue that is troubling the child and put it into a different context from that of his actual life circumstances. For example, with a bed-wetting issue, where a child is feeling full of shame, take the theme into a fantastical context – say a hedgehog in a forest who is dealing with a problem of leaks. This provides the protection of disguise and indirect expression.

The surreal, the fantastical and the absurd all work well when changing the literal into the symbolic: sometimes the more 'dotty' the better. For example, in *Willy and the Wobbly House* (Sunderland & Armstrong, 2000), the fact that Mrs Flop is a very bizarre other-worldly character from the post office, or that Mrs Thumpabot (in *A Nifflenoo Called Nevermind*, Sunderland & Armstrong, 2000) does not stand on her legs, and so on, is fine in the world of the story, just as such absurd things are perfectly accepted by the dreamer in the dream. In choosing a context, think of things, places and characters that children love, such as Disneyland, chocolate, chips, rainbows, fireworks or bouncy castles.

Do not clutter the message in your story with irrelevancies

Pare away all unnecessary detail and wordiness. Abstraction means the process of reducing a thing to its most fundamental identity: the essential characteristics that make it what it is. The story should *abstract* the most important features of the emotional issue that you have chosen, cutting through the superficial or irrelevant. A lot of stories are severely weakened by clutter: too many words, sloppy meanderings into detail or irrelevance. This detracts from the content. A therapeutic story needs to pack its punch, and for that it needs to be succinct. So take away anything that weakens its impact or obscures its meaning or logic. Otherwise, the child may not hear the important psychological message because of all the other meanings and issues that you have brought in.

Some common questions about telling therapeutic stories to children

'What's the youngest age for a child to respond to a therapeutic story?'

Around the age of three. This is because in many ways pre-three-year-olds still live in a very concrete world; their play is still largely about concrete things. They like stories about clearing the house, going swimming, driving a tractor, making a cake or going to the park. They like these stories because they are still at the age of being introduced to such things in the world. And so they like the recognition and revisiting in a book. But from age three, and then very powerfully at four, children start to live vividly in the world of their imaginations.

'But I really don't think I can make up stories on the spot.'

It is fine to go away and think about what story your child would benefit from hearing. Take as long as you need. Then, when you find the right moment with the child, you may want to enact the story with little toys, or to use cartoons or pictures you have drawn. A story with visuals – pictures, or enacted live with toys and figures, or with lots of expressive gestures – will always engage a child far more than just telling it. The more multisensory it is, the more powerfully the story can be evoked.

'But how do I get started? And how can I be sure that I have chosen the right emotional theme for the child?'

One way to find out is to imagine that you have asked the child to draw a picture, or to do a sandplay picture of what it feels like to be him in his life now. Then *you* draw the picture and/or do the sandplay picture you think he would do if he was being very honest and open. In doing this exercise, it means you are listening to the wisdom of your own imagination, rather than just using your thinking self. You may realise, by making your drawing or doing your sandplay, that you have picked up far more things about the child's inner world than you thought.

I followed this process in designing a story for a little boy with whom I was working. He was traumatised from having been beaten up by his father so badly that he was taken into care. In care, although he made some good friends, he was bullied by other boys because he was so frightened and vulnerable. Below is the story I told him. It was born out of my doing a sandplay enactment of what I imagined he would do if he expressed what it felt like to be him. The sandplay picture was informed by my having spent a lot of time with the little boy, as well as having read all the notes on his trauma and seeing how he was with other children and adults, and how he expected them to make him feel small and powerless. In doing the sandplay of his inner world, through including my imagination in the empathic process, I reached a deeper level of understanding of what it must be like to be him. Having done my sandplay picture, I realised that any story I told would have to empathise with the little boy's feelings of terrible aloneness and debilitating fear of feeling overwhelmed in a hostile world; with his feelings of despair, and with the fact that he had all too little concept of getting help or support from kind and concerned others.

The story of Teenie Weenie in the Frightening Forest

Teenie Weenie was a little chicken, who one day found himself, not on a farm, but in some awful undergrowth in a forest. Suddenly, a monkey roared at him and he cowered into a little ball. He walked along a bit more, but then the leaves crackled and he felt even smaller. And then an owl hooted at him and he felt smaller still. And the more Teenie Weenie found the forest too much, the smaller he felt. By the time all manner of creatures had snarled at him, hooted at him, sneered or squawked at him, he felt he was little more than a speck. And because he felt like a speck, the tiniest little insect in the jungle wanted to eat him. So he ran away very fast, and hid. While he was hiding, he realised that he just wanted to give up. 'What's the point of living in such a too-big world?' he thought.

But then along strolled a bird with beautiful feathers. 'Hey, I noticed you hiding there,' he said, and he smiled at Teenie Weenie. 'Why don't you come out of there and have tea with me?' Teenie Weenie said he couldn't. 'It's far too frightening out there in the world.' 'Nonsense,' said the bird, 'If we go together it isn't frightening. I agree that doing

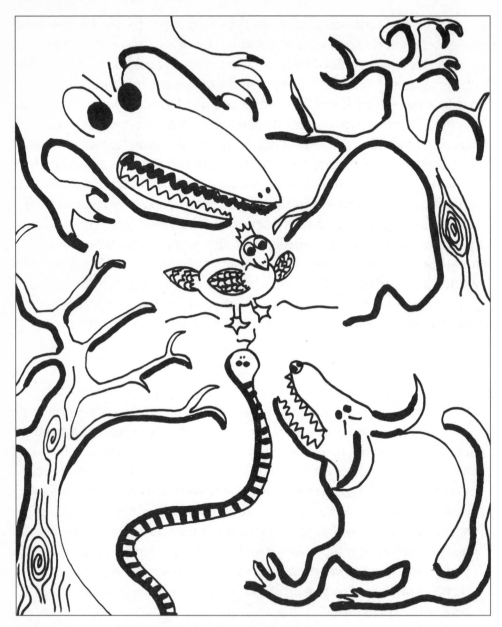

Figure 3 *Teenie Weenie in the frightening forest*

brave things on your own can be far too frightening and far too lonely; but together, it can be fun and interesting. And – guess what! – here is my friend Hedgehog!' So Teenie Weenie, Hedgehog and the beautiful bird all went off together to the beautiful bird's house for tea. And when they met some stinging insects along the way, they all said 'Boo!' together, and so the insects didn't bother them any more. And when the owls tooted, the beautiful bird and Teenie Weenie and Hedgehog hooted back, so the owl said, 'Oh dear, I'll go and hoot somewhere else.' And when a skunk hissed, the three of them together just hissed back so the skunk skunked off. Teenie Weenie had never felt better in his life. He felt all warm inside. And they all had a very nice tea indeed.

And after that day, whenever Teenie Weenie realised that he was starting to shrink, he said to himself 'Oops! I need some help from a friend', and he went and got it. He never forgot how *together* feels so good, and how *all alone* just feels terribly, terribly lonely and frightening, as it makes the world a too difficult place to be. And so from that time Teenie Weenie's life was a far, far better life to live.

'How do I know if a story has got through to a child on a deep level?'

You will sense if a child is absorbed in a story or not. If the child asks, 'Can we have that story again?', the story's message may well have been of real importance to him.

A story as successful therapeutic intervention can also show itself by a child starting to use some of the creative ways of being or coping in the story, in his own life. But he may not do this immediately. It may not be right for him to do this straight away. Rather, the story may plant a seed in his mind that grows into a fully-fledged idea or way of being that he acts on in later life.

A story as successful therapeutic intervention can shift old confusions or set beliefs in the child's mind, such as 'I am stupid', 'I can never be any different', or 'People just don't like me because I am so weak/dull.'

A child may be inspired to write or draw something as a result of the story, meaning that his mind is clearly still processing it.

'Could I tell the child a story about my own life?'

Be careful about this. In hearing painful stories from *your* life, a child can feel burdened, rather than empathised with. If, for example, you say *you* were frightened or sad, children may feel they have to look after you, or that you are not strong enough to look after them. They may think, 'Oh dear, there are no strong adults around me after all. This adult is a frightened little girl underneath just like me. I'd better not show her any of my strong or fierce feelings.' In telling a story about your life, however relevant, you do not know how the child will receive it, and what insecurities he may feel about you and him together as a result. He may feel that he has lost his strong protective ally.

'Could I tell the child a story about another child who was coping with something, like him, and who found a creative way of dealing with it?'

Yes – and it can be a fictitious other child. This is often a powerful way of getting your message across at an unconscious level: 'I knew a little girl once – a bit like you . . . she had this problem . . .' Then again, tell the journey from the problem to crisis to solution. It works because, again, it is an indirect expression and so holds all the power that we have already talked about.

CHAPTER 3

How to Make an Effective Response when a Child Tells a Story to You

HOW CAN A CHILD tell you in everyday language how he feels – when his natural language for feeling is one of story, play and imagination? As we saw in Chapter 1, the language of literal words is not the natural language for children to use to speak about their feelings. Without communication through story, play or imagination, some children have little hope of being able to say what they really feel. Troubled children can be helped immeasurably if someone can hear them speak through story.

In general, children are not good at answering the direct question, 'How are you feeling?' You often get silence, or an inaccurate label such as 'bored' or 'fed up', which can actually mean a myriad things: 'hurt', 'disappointed', 'I feel just awful about myself', 'falling apart', 'feeling like no one wants to play with me', and so on.

Children tend to have a very limited vocabulary to express their feelings (sad, cross, not fair, bored, happy, scared), and yet they feel a hundred other feelings that are not included in this limited list. With such a restricted verbal vocabulary, they tend to select a feeling word that may seem like the feeling they are having, but which is actually quite another. Thus they often fail to reach their listeners in a way that they can really know or understand. How can a parent, teacher or social worker offer a child in-depth empathy, and be able to 'imagine themselves into' the child's world and sensory reality, when that child is speaking in a language of feeling that is not his natural one? In short, without having access to imaginative modes of expression, the deeply rich inner worlds of too many children remain unshared.

To illustrate, the following is an example of a little girl called Cleo who could not speak about her feelings through everyday language, but spoke superbly about them through story.

Cleo, aged seven

Ever since her sister was born, Cleo's schoolwork had gone downhill. At home Cleo appeared more and more angry, and said repeatedly how 'unfair' it was that she couldn't have more sweets, more pocket money, later bedtime, more comics, more clothes, more treacle pudding, and so on. Cleo had put her very complex feelings about her new sister being around into one very little, very inadequate feeling word – 'unfair'. Her parents had not read this as being about her sister at all, and had got increasingly cross with her 'demands'. This was a classic communication breakdown between adult and child.

Luckily, Cleo went to see a child counsellor, as her worsening school achievements were greatly worrying her parents. In counselling, by enacting the following stories through play, Cleo spoke with amazing eloquence about her very complex feelings about her sister, herself and her mother. Through story she could talk about many more feelings than just 'unfair'. In other words, once she had image and metaphor as a language, Cleo spoke about her troubled feeling with real poetic depth.

Cleo's stories enacted through toys in a sandplay:

Story 1 The princess has lost her treasure* to someone else. She sees someone else wearing the tiara she once wore, and it makes her cry.

Story 2 A hedgehog and a toad are fighting over a jewel.* The hedgehog kills the toad for taking the jewel. The hedgehog feels terrible about it. She hadn't meant to kill, it was because she so badly wanted the jewel.

Story 3 The queen puts candles and fruit on the table for the princess, but then at the last minute she gives them to the sweet little kitten instead, because she likes the kitten so much.

Story 4 One night, the princess of thieves robbed the castle, but instead of jewels,* her pockets were full of sand.

Story 5 There is a magic key to a magic place. The bird with broken wings needs the key to get in, but you see it can't get in. Its dream is to get in.

Story 6 The little squirrel lived in a lovely house, but the council came and repossessed it.

Story 7 A princess is dancing with the queen – and the maid is looking at them from the balcony.

Through these stories, Cleo communicated her pain:

Story 1 Feelings of having lost her mother to her sister, and her grief about that.

Story 2 Her wish to wipe out her sister, from a desperate need to get back to Mummy again, and guilt about these feelings.

Story 3 Feeling she is the less preferred, feeling cast aside, and that she cannot light up her mother as her little sister can.

Story 4 The feeling of having metaphorically to steal what she needs: for example, getting her mother's attention by manipulative means. Grumbling about her pocket money is a hollow victory. It might get her mother's attention, but it doesn't win her love.

Story 5 Feeling excluded; feeling locked out of her mother's heart or body, not knowing how to get back in.

Story 6 Cleo probably feels that her sister has 'repossessed' her mother! She feels usurped, left in a state of emotional emptiness.

* *It is very common in children's stories for a jewel or treasure to symbolise the fought-over parent.*

Story 7 The agony of having to 'use your eyes to drink in somebody else's Garden of Eden' (Armstrong-Perlman, 1997).

George fell into a very withdrawn state until a counsellor listened to him speak his feelings through story.

George, aged eight

George was a happy little boy until his mother became very depressed after the sudden death of her own mother. A teacher, seeing George so withdrawn and miserable and knowing his home circumstances, had asked George one day, 'What do you feel about your mother being unhappy?' George had just shrugged his shoulders and moved away. Other teachers and relatives also tried to ask George what he was feeling, and had similarly met a 'keep out!'

Luckily, George went to a school where there was a child counsellor on site, so he agreed to go to see her.

George started by painting a fog. The counsellor asked George to tell her about his picture. George told the following story about it:

'The fog is too thick. I can't stop it getting everywhere. It takes me from the sun and puts me in the dark land. I need to make myself happy so that the fog will lift, but when I try, I breathe in more fog. I struggle and struggle to get it out of me. The trouble is, Mum has swallowed too much fog too.'

Through his story, George spoke most eloquently of his feelings about his mother's depression getting everywhere, affecting him intensely, as if getting right inside him. His story reminded me of CS Lewis's similar, forceful metaphor to describe his grief when his wife died: 'Her absence is like the sky. It spreads over everything' (1966).

With an adult who could hear him speaking through story, George spoke clearly and powerfully. With adults who offered him only everyday language, he just shrugged his shoulders: no connection was possible.

A summary of the benefits for children of telling their feelings through story

To a child, everyday words can feel stale or dry, whereas a story can enable him to be fully there with imagination and feeling. 'Talking about' feeling is rather like spectating life, whereas the process of imagining oneself into feeling through enactment and story is like getting on with being fully involved in life as a player, not a spectator.

Story can enable a child to express the many different meanings and feelings about an experience he has had, *all at the same time*. It can therefore capture a fuller picture of a child's perceptual reality. In so doing, a story can convey a great deal of information, in contrast to reductionist literal statements such as, 'I'm cross' or 'I'm bored.' Feeling words can hide, whereas story can reveal.

It can be an immense relief for a child to find images and metaphors to express his thoughts or feelings which have previously been nameless and yet craved understanding. Everyday words often fail to convey the full qualitative and energetic aspects of what the child is experiencing; the emotional atmosphere of a particular moment or situation. Enacting emotional experience through story, via drawing, clay, movement, puppets or music can enable the child to reach beyond generalising everyday feeling words to a far deeper and more specific truth: 'Art throws off the covers that hide the expressiveness of experienced things' (Dewey, 1934, p104).

As a result of having played out a story, the troubled child often has a sense of, '*Yes*! This is really what I wanted to say', 'I've really let you know now', or 'I have told you exactly what it is like to be me at the moment.' The right language of expression frees the child. The wrong language imprisons him.

In short, for children, story is a communication technique – an extremely potent one.

Trauma and anti-social behaviour

If a traumatised child does not tell the story of his trauma, he may unconsciously act it out through anti-social behaviour. Some troubled children who cause major problems at school, at home or on the streets, are, unconsciously, acting out aspects of *the story* of a trauma they have suffered. Scientific research about trauma and post-traumatic stress shows that repeating the trauma in this way is the mind trying to assimilate it. So, in trauma theory, much bullying in the playground is triggered by the bully's out-of-awareness compulsion to repeat the traumatic things which that happened to him, or that he has witnessed.

When feelings about a trauma are too awful and unbearable, they need to be banished to the unconscious. But it is in the unconscious that they can cause such misery. As Freud said, about repression and the unconscious, 'feelings proliferate [there] in the dark' (1915, p148). Then the repressed emotional energy leaks out in all manner of neurotic symptoms (see Figure 4).

Trauma research also shows how, in acting out an aspect of his trauma, the traumatised child can take the role either of the persecutor or his original victim. (One of the most respected books on trauma research is Van der Kolk *et al*, 1996.) Many bullies in the playground, for example, have been bullied themselves – eg, by a sibling, parent, teacher or relative – but now take the role of the persecutor, and get some other innocent child to be the victim. In this way, they make that other child experience the feelings they themselves felt during the trauma. Sadly, though, because the trauma is repeated without being properly felt and thought through in conscious awareness, usually nothing gets resolved. Rather, the story of the trauma carries on haunting the traumatised child (and his victims). He keeps revisiting the feelings of the trauma in his dreams; in his acting out behaviour, and in his ways of relating to people. Freud called this 'repetition compulsion' (1917), while Van der Kolk has written: 'The trauma keeps them rigidly fixated on the past, making them fight the last battle over and over again' (Van der Kolk, 1989, p17).

This haunting also means that the feelings of the trauma keep getting retriggered. It only need be an image, or a sound, or a certain facial expression and the child is reliving the whole thing again. For example, Billy, aged seven, suffered much physical abuse at the hands of his stepfather. So when any male member of staff looked at him

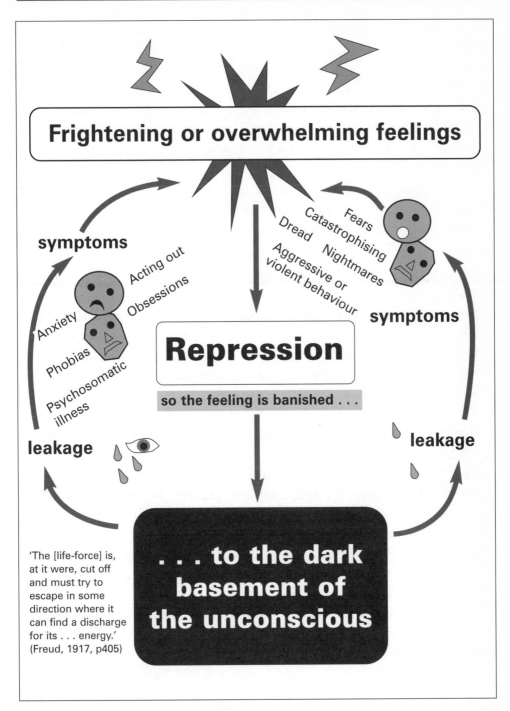

Figure 4 *What neurosis looks like*

crossly he would physically lash out at him. Some would see this as a massive over-reaction, but in terms of trauma theory, Billy's reaction made perfect sense: 'Because people with post-traumatic stress disorder [cannot] integrate traumatic experiences with other life events, their traumatic memories are often not coherent stories; they tend to consist of intense emotions or somatosensory impressions, which occur when the victims are aroused or exposed to reminders of the trauma' (Van der Kolk *et al*, 1996, p9).

An example of a traumatised child re-enacting the story of her trauma, but out of her conscious awareness

This little girl had been in an awful accident when she was a toddler – a truck careered into her at a bus stop. She could not deal with her feelings about it. They were too awful. So she forgot it all, and banished the memory of it to her unconscious. However, when she went to school, she would rush into a group of children and knock them down. Otherwise she was well behaved. She was enacting the trauma, but this time with herself as the persecutor – the truck! (Cited in Share, 1994, p56.)

But if children have the opportunity to tell the story of their trauma, to someone who can really listen and help them work through their feelings about it, they will not need to keep acting out parts of the story of that trauma in anti-social ways. This 'trauma storytelling' needs to be done in the presence of an empathic adult who will help the child properly process the trauma, so his mind can finally put it to rest, and he can get on with his life without being haunted by it. Story provides time for conscious reflection of traumatic feelings, rather than just discharging them (for example, over other children in the playground). Dewey says of art, but it applies just as well to story, that it 'takes the indirect road of expression instead of the direct road of discharge' (1934, p78).

Stories traumatised children have told as a vital part of processing their feelings

Before they had access to storytelling, the children below enacted their trauma in antisocial ways. But when they could tell it through story, their antisocial behaviour stopped.

Eddie, aged seven

Eddie had seen his father attack his mother on several occasions. It was so awful that he chose to 'forget' the experience. But from the age of four onwards, he became an awful bully in the playground. On one occasion he kept pushing a little girl's head down into the gravel. He was enacting the story of his trauma. The following are Eddie's stories in counselling, enacted through play:

'The policeman, fireman, doctor, lollipop lady all die and the dustbin man is left to shovel them up.'
(Translation: here, the protectors – all the adults who are supposed to help – are rendered impotent. Eddie has suffered the awful pain of no one helping him and no one helping his mother while he watched his father beat her up.)

'People are scared of the dragon. The dragon smashes up people's houses, that's why they hate him.'
(Translation: he fears and hates his father's violence.)

'Children are battling with things in the underworld. They are just battling and battling and battling. There is never an end to the battling.'
(Translation: every time Eddie hits a little girl he is showing he is battling with awful memories in his head. The underworld is a common image for the unconscious.)

'The little worm cries, "Mummy Mummy, there's a big crow!" The little worm is calling for its Mummy, but the Mummy worm just runs away frightened, too. The Mummy worm ends up being eaten by the big crow. Lots of things are crawling on her grave.'
(Translation: he wanted Mummy to save him from seeing the awful scene, but she can't help him because she herself is being attacked and

frightened. The bit about crawling on her grave may be his feelings of disgust about what he saw, but it is difficult to say.)

'This is a story about a cruel garden. The big tree whacks the little tree, so that there are no flowers on it next year. All the daisies watched. They wanted to stop it from happening, but they were too small to do anything.'
(Translation: the pain of himself as the impotent watcher.)

After all these stories in metaphor, one day Eddie told his counsellor about the actual events of the trauma. And yet he still talked poetically and with metaphor. Here are some of the things he said:

'I was very, very scared, like when you go down the water-chute in the swimming pool and your face smacks the water.'
'People don't think when they fight.'
'I only have one feeling – it's called muddledy-mess.'
(Translation: how can he make sense of all this? He loved his father and yet saw him hitting his mother.)

Sarah, aged six

Sarah had also witnessed parental violence and had been beaten on several occasions by her father. She was subsequently so aggressive and hostile in school that no one wanted to be her friend. The following are Sarah's stories in counselling, enacted through play:

'There are sleeping horrible things. We mustn't wake them.'
'The king is burning babies in the fire. He doesn't realise what he is doing. A woman gets touched by the fire. It blew up and killed her too.'
(Translation: the horror of the out-of-control fiery passion of her father which has burnt both herself and her mother.)

'The crow flew right into the king's head and took away his kindness, so that he didn't remember his kindness.'
(Translation: when father is hitting, he loses all his humanity. He is as if possessed.)

'The only safe place is on top of a mountain. Then a man leaps on the mountain and attacks everyone.'
(Translation: the place that is meant to be safe is unsafe.)

To her counsellor: 'I want to throw you into the smelly, rat-infested dungeon'; 'You've got to punish me'; 'I want you to shout at me, it makes me feel better than when you are kind to me.'
(Translation: she is enacting in the therapeutic relationship the type of cruel power-based relationships she witnessed so often at home.)

Both Eddie's and Sarah's counsellors were able to empathise with the horror and pain in these stories, while staying within the metaphor. They were able to feed back 'message received and understood' about the feelings of impotence, frustration, confusion, fear, hate, desperate unsafety, aloneness and so on. As a result, Eddie stopped beating up little girls at school and Sarah started to make friends. Their counsellors had heard and understood their stories, so they no longer needed to act them out (unconsciously) in antisocial ways. They were no longer haunted by what they had experienced.

I end this section with two other examples of acting-out behaviour, and how much of it is communication through story and metaphor, if you take the time and trouble to read it.

Terry, aged twelve

Terry felt traumatically 'let down' by his father, who put him into care after the death of his mother. Terry's residential care worker said he would buy him a MacDonalds for his birthday. He forgot. That evening Terry 'let down' his social worker's tyres.

Susan, aged fifteen

In a residential care home, Susan was telling her mother excitedly how she was in love with a boy for the first time in her life. Her mother called her a dirty little slut. Susan put the phone down and went and pulled up all the flowers in the garden. Although this was, of course, a destructive act, it is a highly understandable metaphorical communication for a teenager who felt that her mother had just 'pulled up' and damaged her delight in her flowering loving feelings, flowering sexuality and flowering relationship.

Resources needed for a child to play out a story

Many children under the age of ten can communicate through story with as little as a few paper tissues, toilet-roll middles, the odd egg-carton and a few miniature figures. So with this age group, if you are worried that you do not have enough toys, paints, clay and so on, it can often be that you are actually worrying about whether you have enough 'emotional resources' to offer the child, rather than a lack of toys.

I remember my five-year-old niece when we were both attending a formal golden wedding lunch. I was thinking, 'Damn! I've forgotten to bring any toys. How is Emily going to be able to last for three hours with no means of play?' But in two minutes Emily pointed with glee at a knife and a fork she had tucked up in a napkin: 'Look, two people in bed!' She then went into an elaborate story (which lasted for a good part of the lunch), about them living in a secret magical world underneath the tablecloth.

However, some children have been too discouraged in the realm of imaginative play to be able to react like this, and so they do need more actual toys to support their journey into imaginary worlds. Ideally, what you need in the room to inspire a child to tell a story is a sandbox. This is usually about 23 × 29 × 3 inches (57 × 72 × 7 cm). It should be painted blue on the bottom to represent water and then filled with sand. Children use the sandbox as their theatre. It is the frame or forum for the action in the story. Of course, a story can take place on the floor or via a drawing, but lots of children like the three-dimensional environment of the sandbox. Because of the sand, you can bury things or bomb things, and everything stands up easily. When you wet the sand you can mould it into a fort, an island, a cave and so on, so the little miniatures can be given an immediate environment or stage, all set for the action of the story.

Many child workers who use sandplay have a big choice of toy miniatures, aiming to represent most key objects in the world. This is one reason why sandplay therapy is known as 'the world technique' (see Lowenfeld, 1991, for more on sandplay therapy). I started off with about 20 miniatures, and the children I worked with made up excellent stories. The important thing is to have some miniatures from each of the following categories:

- Transport (must include emergency service vehicles) as well as train, aeroplane, helicopter, car, bus and so on
- People (to include figures of aggression or cruelty and figures of love or warmth; mythical figures such as trolls, witches and fairies; family members)
- People in professions (for example, policeman, nurse, lollipop lady, teacher)
- Monsters
- Farmyard animals
- Jungle animals
- Buildings (houses, prison, fort and so on)
- Furniture (bath, bed, armchair, toilet) and food
- Outside man-made world (for example, gate, road, fence)
- Outside natural world (trees, flowers, hedge, stones, shells, cliffs).

How to get a child started in using sandplay for story or enactment

Show the child the miniatures and the sandbox. Put your hands in the sandbox to show the blue on the bottom for water, and how you can wet, then mould the sand into a building, a wall or a dam, and so on, so you have a setting. Show him how you can then put miniatures in the setting to make up a story, or a play or a film set. Sandplay can be a very powerful medium for storytelling, following are some examples.

Figure 5 (page 44) is a drawing of a sandplay story told by a ten-year-old girl. She called it 'The Cave of Bad Mothers and Dead Babies'. The girl had been beaten by her mother on many occasions, and had to be taken into care. The girl's therapist empathised with what a terrible place the

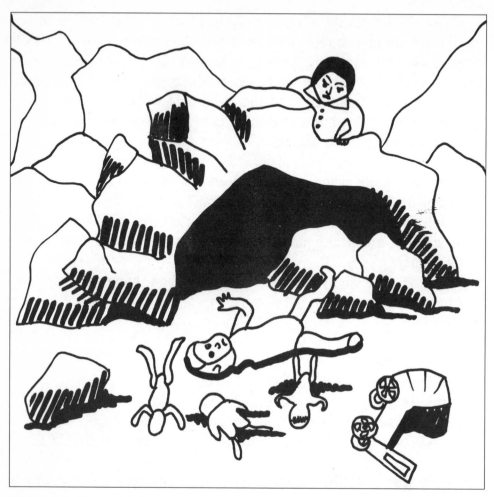

Figure 5 *The cave of bad mothers and dead babies*

cave was, and how terrifying for the babies, who had no one there to protect them; and how the mothers in the story, who were supposed to be the ones protecting the babies, were actually frightening them to death. The child's communication with her therapist was all done in metaphor. If she had wanted to say what had happened to her overtly, she would have done so. Later in the therapy, the girl did talk directly about her physical abuse, saying, 'I felt like I had died many times.'

Figure 6 depicts a sandplay story told by an eight-year-old boy who had actually thrown himself off a bridge, but had survived. His story was

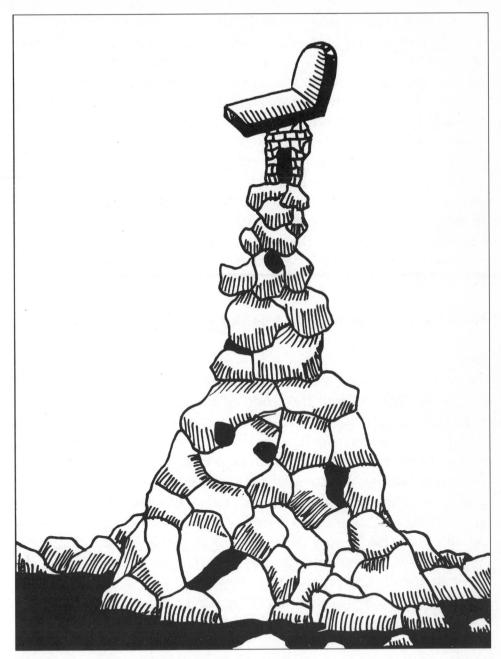

Figure 6 *The grave at the top of the mountain*

about a little old man who was so sad that he wanted to live on his own – far, far away from people – on the top of a mountain. But the only place he could find to live there was a gravestone. No one knew he was there and, because the mountain was so steep, no one could be bothered to find him. It is a terribly desolate and heartbreaking story, showing that this little boy's inner world was truly bleak and lacking in all comfort, warmth and feelings of being wanted.

In his life, the little boy was indeed in a place of despair, as his mother said that she could no longer manage him, and so he was put into care. He would run away from the children's home and hide in his mother's garden so as to catch just a glimpse of her through her kitchen window. In the picture taken from the story, you can see how he has perched a symbol of death so precariously on top of the mountain.

How to listen as a child speaks to you through story

Dos

The central task of any counsellor, teacher or social worker is to imagine themselves into the world of the child's story, and then to reflect on that world. What would you feel, being there? Would you be lonely and hopeless, or happy and comforted? Are you in a bleak or malign world, or a benign one with hope of help and comfort? You can do a great deal just by 'imagining yourself in' like this.

Aim to show your interest and emotional resonance by using appropriate vocal sounds, as a kind of Greek chorus comment on the action of the child's story. This is a way of validating the child's ebb and flow of emotional energies and feeling tones in his telling of the story. Be aware, however, that for some children this may get in the way rather than be a useful mirroring. One child did a puppet story which she wanted me to watch. I did the usual Greek chorus sounds. She then wanted to video the puppet story for her mother. On it, of course, were all my oohs and aahs. She turned to her mother and said, 'Mummy, those strange noises in the background are Margot going ooh and ahh. She needs to do that!' The little girl was giving me excellent advice that she really didn't need my oohs and aahs. They were a kind of irrelevant oddity to her!

Don'ts

When listening to children's feelings as told to you through story or through everyday language, a number of pitfalls must be avoided. Do not offer an uninterested or low-key response to something very central and important to the child. A tepid response when the child is showing an intensity of feeling, such as love, excitement, anger or joy can easily bring blight to a child's natural expressiveness. When you are expecting someone to be sharing your intense experience, it is just too lonely to find that you are actually on your own with it, and that the listening other is just being there in a faded, preoccupied or dutiful way. At best it is embarrassing. At worst it is shaming. Moreover, feeling shamed means a child can all too easily respond by closing down his spontaneity and expressiveness for fear of being shamed again.

Avoid making judgements or giving advice instead of listening and taking the time to imagine yourself into the child's story world and the feeling states presented there. Similarly, avoid taking over what the child is doing or saying in his story. For example, the listening adult may say: 'No, don't leave the little peanut in the gutter – let's get it a nice home to go to.' This is an example of the adult's need to make everything all right, when maybe by leaving the peanut in the gutter the child is trying to communicate his feelings of hopelessness. This is a common problem when the adult listener (usually out of conscious awareness) is running away from her own hopelessness, despair, grief and so on, and so needs to make the child's stories all nice, with nice happy feelings and nice happy endings. The paradox for the hopeless child is that there is much hope in being able to find someone who can really hear and be with their hopelessness.

Do noT attempt to talk a child out of his feelings, saying for example, 'No, you shouldn't feel like that', or 'it's silly to think that!' Stay with a child's feeling, rather than subtly or unsubtly trying to persuade him to have a different one. You may be finding the feelings he is having difficult because of your own emotional blocks. This may cause you to justify to yourself why it is a good idea to get him to feel something other than what he is expressing in his story.

Do not follow your interest about some aspect of the child's story, or what you see in the sandbox or drawing, rather than following theirs: 'Ah, I see, so the fox eats the chickens. But I'm very interested in the pink blancmange you've drawn in the corner of your picture. Tell me about that now.' At that particular moment the child was very much with the fox and the chickens, yet the listener has let his own curiosity interrupt. This gives the message to the child, 'I'm not really listening to what you are saying here about the fox and the chickens.'

Beware your own unconscious 'deafness' or 'blindness'. If you are defending yourself against feeling some of your own very painful emotions, such as despair, hopelessness, fear or anger, you may not be able to hear these feelings in a child's stories. You *listen*, but do not *hear*. This is because no one has helped *you* fully feel and think about these painful feelings in yourself. If you have repressed certain painful feelings from your own childhood, and the child expresses these same feelings in his story, you are likely to be blind to them – and blind to the fact that you are blind to them. This is because, as we have said, repression is a defence, which means that you have forgotten that you have forgotten. (This is why a compulsory part of a child counsellor's or therapist's training is their own therapy – to ensure that their own emotional blocks do not block the child.)

If you have emotional blocks like this, children tend to become aware of them and then they stop wanting to tell you stories with certain emotional themes. Rather, they may say, 'Let's play football', or, 'Let's play chess', or something similar. And if your blocks get in the way too often, children may shut you out of their feeling life entirely. They feel too unsafe to go on the journey into painful emotional processing with you, because they know that, in very important ways, you will not be there with them. Consequently, the journey will be too lonely. If you are working therapeutically with children and this keeps happening, it is an indication that it is time to get therapy, or more therapy, for yourself.

Imagining yourself into a child's story and the psychological landscape being presented

Avoid making deductions from a 'one-off' story. It is the recurrent theme and recurrent psychological landscape that presents the clearest picture of the child's inner world. So the child who repeatedly presents warm, friendly worlds in his stories, or who repeatedly presents hostile, cold ones, is telling you a lot about the state of his inner world: his world of feelings, beliefs, images, sensations, emotionally charged memories, and particular sense of self and of others.

Perception of the outer world is always hugely coloured by our inner world. In fact, neurobiologically speaking, perception is always filtered through memory, although by and large we are not aware that this is happening. So when interacting with outer reality, we are constantly registering all events on an inner-world level. This is why a child can be terrified of all men with moustaches because once he had a very frightening teacher who had a moustache. It is this inner-world colouring which means that different people will register the same event very differently. This is why a very depressed child can be taken to a most beautiful place and still feel depressed. In his depression, his inner world is far stronger than his outer-world reality. Whereas a child who feels deeply loved can be in raptures over being taken to a little coffee shop and being given a chocolate muffin. The latter child finds it exquisitely beautiful because he is there with his mother whom he loves.

'People live simultaneously in an external and an internal world and the relationship between the two ranges from the most fluid intermingling to the most rigid separation' (Greenberg & Mitchell, 1987, p68). A child's story can often present a vivid picture of his inner world, as the following example shows:

Pippa, aged seven

Pippa has seen some horrid things happen at home (external reality), and yet she knows that basically she loves her mother very much and that her mother loves her very much (there is therefore an 'inner wealth' in her inner world, as described by the psychoanalyst Melanie Klein).

So Pippa did stories of some awful things happening (external world reality), and yet in her stories there were also images of warmth and comfort, and the most beautiful of treasure (inner world reality).

Edwin, aged nine

Edwin is a child from a nice, middle-class background where there is no abuse or trauma going on whatsoever (outer world), and yet his stories in the classroom are always of bleak places with very lonely people (inner world). His connection to both his workaholic parents is often one of emotional distance, and it transpired in therapy that he did not feel enjoyed or cherished by either of them (inner world).

There are many features to look out for in the psychological landscape of a child's story – including some that are conspicuous by their absence. Images that suggest a harsh, hostile or bleak inner world include the following:

- Images of isolation: desert, wilderness, banishment, exile, on the outside looking in
- Images of aggression, attack and harm: characters symbolising cruelty or persecution
- Images of domination: characters seeking power over the innocent or the helpless, with a total lack of concern and empathy
- Images of fighting: battlefields, bleeding, killing, death
- Images of brutal punishment, or ruthless condemnation without fair trial
- Images of powerlessness or helplessness
- Images of people who are supposed to help, rendered impotent (for example emergency services rendered impotent – typically, something happens to them on their way to helping, so they never reach the victim)
- Images of neglect, decay (often a metaphor for emotional neglect)
- Images of ruin
- Images of burning, fire or flood (often a metaphor for something overwhelming, unmanageable, too intense in oneself or someone else);

- Images of catastrophe or disaster
- Images of damage beyond repair
- Images of brokenness: cracks, things in bits, shards, something that has fallen apart (often a metaphor for broken connections with someone important, or feelings of being broken inside)
- Images of emptiness, scarcity, insufficiency or starvation (often a metaphor for emotional hunger or starvation)
- Images of 'lack' (such as windows without curtains, beds without blankets, pets without owners. Often a metaphor for emotional neglect or emotional hunger).

Absences – what is *not* there in the story's psychological landscape is as important as what *is* there:

- Absence of things growing, such as greenness, foliage, flowers, trees
- Absence of images of shelter, safety, home, sanctuary
- Absence of warm, loving characters
- Absence of human kindness or concern
- Absence of gentleness
- Absence of cosiness or comfort
- Absence of friends
- Absence of potent help, protectors
- Absence of any strong, warm human connection between any of the characters
- Absence of wit or humour.

Figure 7 (page 52) is a drawing of a sandplay story of a child's harsh psychological landscape. This was done by Peter, aged six. It is a story about being attacked by every sort of monster and fierce animal, who are also attacking each other. He said, 'If you were there you wouldn't survive.' Both Peter's parents were drug addicts. He said he did not feel loved by them.

Psychological landscapes may also include images that suggest something good, warm, rich or comforting in the child's inner world.

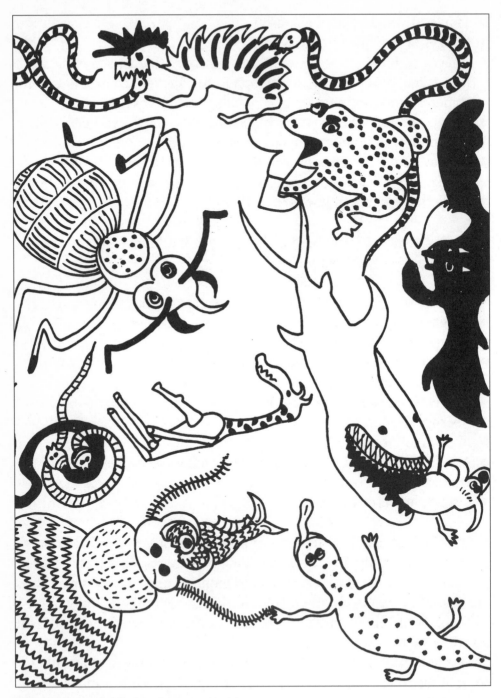

Figure 7 *A child's harsh inner world*

Images such as the following may only appear at some point during the story:

- An overall sense of ease, safety, emotional warmth
- Cosiness
- Beauty
- Kindness
- Hope
- Images of home, or of 'at-homeness' in oneself
- Images of soothing
- Images of calm
- Images of fun
- Images of concern
- Images of there being enough, of abundance or of richness in some form or other
- Images of nourishment (as a symbol of emotional nourishment)
- Interactions between characters which are encouraging and warm
- Interactions between characters which have a sense of 'Yes we can', 'Together we can'.

The objection might be voiced, 'But if a child does a "happy, happy" story, maybe it is just wishful thinking?' Indeed it may be. However, I would argue that, for a child to even conceive of a benign world, he will, at some time in his life, have had first-hand experience of it. So much so, that it is now an active resource in his inner world (even if, at this time in his life, there is little evidence of it in his outer reality). Children who have consistently known a very harsh outer reality without sufficiently powerful relational experiences of human kindness, love, warmth and so on will not be able to imagine such a benign place. Consequently, they will not be able to make up a story about it.

Figure 8 represents a story told by a child who fundamentally had a benign inner world. Gemma, aged five, told the story through miniature figures in a sandbox about a little girl who was frightened of the dark. She enacted in the story some very kind people, saying 'Never mind little girl, here is a light and here is a teddy bear. We will make you safe, so that you are not frightened of the dark! You can call

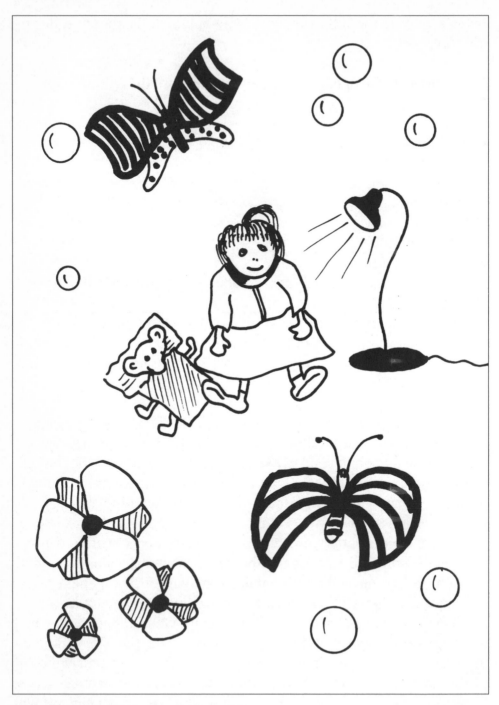

Figure 8 *A child's benign inner world*

out at any time and we will come.' See the images here of comfort, kindness and tenderness.

Through the story, Gemma was working through and rehearsing managing her feelings of fear of the dark, and calling on resources of concern and kindness in her *inner* world to help her.

'An inner world . . . can be rich or poor and can be at peace or in a state of war.' (Winnicott, 1951 quoted in Davis & Wallbridge, 1981, p30).

Looking at central emotional themes rather than detail and meaning of individual images

Look at this story told by an 11-year-old girl called Sophie. Sophie was sexually abused as a child. At first glance you may think, 'There is no way I can understand this story' – but without looking at the answer below, try to find the recurrent central emotional themes in her story. Use the list on pages 23–24 to help you. What feelings about her trauma do you think Sophie is trying to communicate and process in this story? Remember: avoid getting hooked on detail.

Sophie's story

'A bomb is being dropped on an egg, so that the egg can't hatch, and then the tortoise steps on a pea and it gets squashed into the pavement for the next five years. Then the tortoise chews up a little mouse and spits it out half-alive, and a pizza is flying about in the air and hits an old man on the nose. And people are trapped in a bus shelter and they call for help, but that just makes the roof fly off the bus shelter, so they are not safe any more. Then the sky fills with soot and slime and it pours down on them, so they get drowned in it and their clothes are all smeared by it. However hard they try, they can't get it off them. And then all the crisp-packets explode in the supermarket and so the supermarket falls down and crushes the customers.'

Answer

A bomb is being dropped on the egg, so that the egg can't hatch and then the tortoise steps on a pea and it gets squashed into the pavement for the next five years (themes: abused, powerless, insignificant, trapped. Think of the power differential between a bomb and an egg, between a tortoise and a pea). Then the tortoise chews up a little mouse and spits it out half-alive (themes: 'rubbished', used and abused) and a pizza is flying about in the air and hits an old man on the nose (theme: abused, powerless). And people are trapped in a bus shelter and they call for help (theme: trapped), but that just makes the roof fly off the bus shelter, so they are not safe any more (theme: feeling of there being nothing or no one safe, feeling powerless). Then the sky fills with soot and slime and it pours down on them, so they get drowned in it and their clothes are all smeared by it. However hard they try, they can't get it off them (theme: invaded, contaminated). And then all the crisp-packets explode in the supermarket, and so the supermarket falls down and crushes the customers (theme: feelings of being destroyed).

How did you get on? (Be reassured! Most stories told be children are not as difficult and dense as this.) The story vividly and repeatedly speaks of Sophie's terrifying feelings of being trapped, powerless, insignificant, abused, 'rubbished', invaded, contaminated and destroyed. Imagine what you would feel if you spent a day in Sophie's story world. Mad probably, and totally alone. The world she presents is brutal and ruthless. It has no kindness, no help, no comfort or concern. It is a very dangerous and unpredictable world where there is no safety. If Sophie had told you this story, she would need to know that you had understood her communication of this living hell on earth, and that you could find the words to convey this empathy to her.

An emotional theme that comes up again and again in a child's stories is clear evidence that he is very busy with that theme, and trying to process and digest it. Where there is a recurring theme, you can draw the child's attention to it. For example: 'I loved your story about the egg that got stuck for ever and ever in the egg-cup. And I was remembering what you did last week – when Frankie got stuck down a dark hole and how he just gave up in there. And the week before that, when the little pig couldn't get out of the ditch [picking up on the recurrent themes of 'stuckness', being trapped, impotence, hopelessness and so on] . . . And I'm thinking, how awful to be so stuck like that, like the egg, and Frankie, and the pig.

How far too lonely and frightening for them all. And I'm thinking that, in your stories, none of them cried out for help. Maybe it just didn't occur to them, or maybe they didn't trust that any help would come. Or maybe they felt that help wouldn't be any good if it did come, I wonder?'

How to respond empathically to the child's story while staying within the metaphor

If a child has chosen the language of metaphor for his story, it is important that you can respond within that language. Many children will tell you all *within the metaphor of a story*. As we have said, metaphor is a child's natural language for feeling. But if, in your response to his story, you come out of the metaphor at the wrong time, he may close down and shut you out of his feeling world. The danger is that, as you have switched languages from the metaphorical to the real, he may stop talking to you even in metaphor.

For example, if, in response to a child's story about cruel farm animals who attack a little dog then shut him in a shed, you come out of metaphor and say something like, 'I wonder if that big pig is what you feel about your Daddy when he hits you', (a) you may be just plain wrong – so the child feels grossly misunderstood, or (b) if the child had wanted a straight conversation about Daddy hitting him, he would have had one. It does no one any good to be prised open in this way. It just means that now the child has to deal with his feelings of being prised open, on top of whatever he was feeling before. That is why speaking through story and metaphor is so good, because it is *indirect* communication. Responding with metaphor is a safe way of ensuring that you respect a child's defences.

So, as a rule, stay within the metaphor as much as you can; empathise with the child within this language, saying, for example, 'How lonely for the little dog there all on his own.' Therapeutic change can happen entirely through the language of metaphor, without your ever referring directly to reality. This is because a major part of therapeutic change is the result of empathy. And you can empathise just as easily with the child's feelings as expressed through metaphor as you can if they were expressed in everyday language. However, if the child ventures information – actively wants to tell you something about his outer life *without* metaphorical coding – fine. Furthermore, I am not saying that you should never come out of metaphor. If you are skilled, you will catch that rare moment when it will be right to comment on how a metaphorically coded part of the child's story reminds you of an aspect of the child's life. But if the child does not take this up, or experiences your switch of language as an interruption – as an invasion – you should drop it and go back to the metaphor.

The situation is somewhat different with children over about ten, and with adolescents. This age-group tends to move from speaking in metaphor in one session to telling you something about their life in literal terms in the next. But again, it is usually best to follow their shift from metaphorical language to literal language and back, rather than you making the shift.

Track the child's story and play, rather than pulling it in the direction you want it to go

You may think you are being helpful, educative and supportive by giving the child new directions for his story. Yet, in fact, you may be quietly suffocating the child's own meaning, his sense of what is of central importance in his story. The following typical examples show adult-led, as opposed to child-led, story and play. Just as the child starts to engage with a toy or an idea in the way he wants, the adult listener comes in with her own ideas about what the child should do next:

- 'No, don't make the little girl drown. See, here is a boat for her.'
- 'No, I think we should look at this bit in your story, not that bit.'
- 'No, don't use that figure, you need a nice kind one. Here's one!'
- 'No, don't feel like that. There really is a lot of hope, you know!'
- 'You're spending so long in that gloomy cave, let's go on to this sunny bit now.'
- 'No, don't leave that bit of the story unfinished – here's a good way to wrap it up.'

If you watch a child enacting something through story in the presence of a directive adult as described here – an adult who offers 'adult-led' as opposed to 'child-led' play – you will often see the child's interest and aliveness fading before your eyes. He stops telling his story and moves on to something else. Either that or he gets cross and becomes rebellious or destructive (banging or smashing things out of frustration, rather than building or constructing things). He has been upstaged by the adult, who has changed his child-led play into adult-led play. The images and characters in his story are robbed of the meaning *he* has given them. Now that his images and characters are imbued with the adult's meaning, they are useless to him.

In short, if the child is fascinated by the long blue line in his story-drawing, and you are fascinated by the old lady he has drawn walking on a cloud at the bottom of the picture, *stay with the long blue line*. This is where the child's energy is. Avoid your own curiosity. Do not let your need to know interrupt what this child is saying or wanting to do. You may refer to the presence of the old lady at some time, but if the child does not pick up your cue – let it go.

The vocabulary to use in your empathic response

An empathic response from the listener is an essential part of the child being enabled to process and work through his feelings about a troubling situation in his inner and/or his outer world. When empathising, make sure your emotional vocabulary is sufficiently rich. If you think only in terms of 'sad', 'angry', 'scared' and 'happy', you may miss a great many of the child's communications via his story, which are about far more complex or more subtle forms of feeling. You may end up trying to put what you see in his story into just one of these four 'feeling words'. With troubled children, you need to be thinking of at least the following list of feelings, in offering an empathic response to the child's story:

- All alone
- Not wanted, or feeling not wanted
- Not enough/never enough
- Horrid inside
- Annoyed

- Not belonging
- Left out
- Missing someone/missing someone so much that it hurts terribly
- Needing something or someone too much
- Hating
- Cross/very cross/very, very cross, not just a bit cross
- Lonely/too lonely
- Unfair
- What's the point of anything (adult version: despair, hopelessness, defeat)
- Desperate
- Confused
- Wobbly inside/too wobbly inside
- Like you are all in bits
- Stuck
- Like you are a nothing
- Like lots of fighting inside your head
- Like you might burst or explode
- Like giving up
- Don't care
- Hurt/very hurt/too hurt
- Disappointed/terribly disappointed
- It's all just too hard
- Too much hurting inside/too much pain inside
- Panic
- Very, very frightened

For example, the counsellor may say (staying with the metaphor), 'I'm thinking about that little dog in your story who fell into the deep, deep well, and how no one heard his cries. So now he just sits there all glum. I'm thinking how all alone he is and how desperate he was to be heard. But now he feels like giving up. It is just too hard.'

Reading poetry is a very good way of enriching your own emotional vocabulary, in order to offer more sensitive and finely-tuned empathic responses to a child's story. Poetry also enables you to respond at times to the child's metaphor with a metaphor of your own. One thing you can say is, 'Your story reminds me of x story or y poem.' If this is helpful to the child, he will run with it in some way, refer to it again, take it into another story. If it isn't, he won't.

By way of example, one therapist quoted from *The Ancient Mariner* in response to the story of her nine-year-old client. This little boy's Daddy had just died, and he was telling a story about a little hedgehog who had lots of kind, loving other hedgehogs in his life who offered him lots of lovely nuts, but he was feeling very hungry and empty and very lonely because he could not eat their food or take their love – he could only take it from someone who wasn't there any more. On hearing and seeing his story, the therapist said to him, 'Water, water everywhere and not a drop to drink.' The little boy looked at her with relief. He clearly felt she had deeply understood his story.

The danger and damage of closed meanings

Never respond by putting your meaning on to a child's image with far too little evidence about what that image means for the child. Although many psychological and dream dictionaries try to define what a certain image means in reality, what, say, a snake means to one child may be something entirely different for another. For one child, a snake may mean a creature who is slowly plotting a sinister death; to another it may be like a large colourful worm, and have no such frightening association whatsoever.

In listening to a child's story, the danger many people fall into is playing 'psychoanalyst', by using closed meanings. For example, a snake means a penis, a sand mound means a breast, a little person between a man and a woman always means a child is wanting to split up Mummy and Daddy. Such interpretation is always dangerous.

It is, of course, tempting to use this apparent short-cut to understanding a child's story (just think, all those useful dream dictionaries available). But it is damaging to *anyone,* not only a child, to be *told* what he feels or thinks, when it is not what he feels and thinks at all. It can be experienced as a psychological assault, an attack or attempted erasing of his own sense of self, meaning and reality. It is turning his story into your story. It is the surest way to make a child stop wanting to tell you anything that really matters to him. The child thinks something like, 'Well here's an adult who can't listen to what I am feeling, and just tells me what I am feeling. It's certainly no good bringing my feelings to her.' Soon there are no more stories, and the child says, 'Can we play football?' The trust is broken and you are unlikely to win it back easily, if at all. So never assume that you know what something means to a child. It may mean something seemingly obvious to you, while actually meaning something entirely different to the child. In short, it is most important always to be sure of the child's meaning for a certain image, character or event in his story, before you offer an empathic response. This is such a crucial point in responding to a child's story that the next section is designed to make this point really clear.

How to recognise when you are responding to a child's story with closed meanings or incorrect interpretations

Many people say, 'But *I* wouldn't interpret', and yet projecting one's own meanings on to the child's image is so easily done, out of awareness. Or rather you may not be admitting that you are making assumptions, without checking first that your meaning for an image in the child's story is the one the child intended.

Some safeguards

Watch out for occasions when your so-called 'observations' are actually incorrect interpretations. For example, a child, enacting his story in the sandpit, says, 'This is a story about a monster, so the giraffe goes flying off, and his friend the sheep is buried in the sand.' The child has given no indication of the feeling content for these images.

Counsellor: 'Ooh, buried – how awful – it must feel terrible in there.' This is the counsellor's assumption. She herself might feel awful if she were buried like the sheep. So get more information from the child, by asking, for example, 'I'm wondering what the sheep feels down there?' (To one child it may mean something like drowning, or being trapped or killed; for another it may mean quite the opposite – somewhere safe, in hiding from the monster.) If the child needs more from you in your question, you can ask, 'Is being buried a good thing for the sheep, or a bad thing?' and then proceed from there:

Child: 'Good.'

Counsellor: 'And it's good because . . .?' (Then the child just has to fill in the end of the sentence.)

Child: 'Because that way he can't get eaten by the monster. The monster will never ever find him there.'

The counsellor can then empathise. She now has enough information about what the 'sheep-being-buried event' means to the child.

Counsellor: 'Phew! It must be a real relief for the sheep that he can find somewhere safe, a place where the monster won't find him.'

So, before you empathise, if you are at all unsure about the meaning of an image, an event or a character for the child, ask him for more information. Never assume.

In the next example, the child tells a story of an angry pig who hates little bees.

Counsellor: 'I think the cross green pig in your story is probably what you are feeling when you see your Mummy smile at the new baby.' (Incorrect and potentially damaging interpretation, the result of not checking information with the child.)

Counsellor (correctly wondering): 'I loved your story. It made me wonder what the green pig was so cross about and what was making him hate little bees so much?'

Other examples of damaging interpretations: a child with an alcoholic mother buries a little blue door in the sand, right at the bottom. One interpretative counsellor may think, 'Aha! This means the child feels swamped by her mother's alcoholism.' Another interpretative counsellor may think, 'Aha, burying . . . this means that the child wants to hide from her mother's problem.' Such thoughts are all likely to be projections, in the sense that maybe the second counsellor wants to hide from something in her own life, or the first therapist feels swamped by something in her life. So, simply ask the child, 'What is it like for the blue door being buried so far down?'

Watch out for hidden incorrect assumptions in the choice of words you use in response to the child's story, as in the following examples:

Child: 'This is a story about a forest. It's got lots of big trees and a path.'

Counsellor: 'Where is the path leading?' The counsellor has brought in the concept of leading, not the child. (The path may not be leading anywhere!)

Counsellor: 'Tell me about that sad cat in your drawing.' (The counsellor has brought in the concept of sad. Maybe she herself is feeling sad today. The cat may be just taking in the view. The child has not given any indication of the cat being sad.)

Counsellor: 'Tell me about the drooping hat.' (The adjective 'drooping' is the counsellor's word. The hat may look droopy to the counsellor, but it may not be perceived as such by the child, or, if it is, it may be an irrelevant aspect of the hat to the child.)

But of course it is possible to get too self-conscious about language: for example, if a child picks up a toy pig and puts it in her story and you think, 'What if the pig isn't a pig, maybe I should not use the word "pig" in my questions, maybe I should just refer to "it"?' So you get worried about not assuming anything about the child's nouns as well, and then you end up feeling completely tongue-tied. Basically, nouns are usually OK. It is only occasionally that a child will need to correct you on a noun; usually this happens with pre-five-year-olds. For example, Stella, aged three, had placed a boat on a plate in the sandtray. The counsellor said, 'Oh, a boat on a plate', but Stella replied, 'It's not a boat – it's an egg and bacon breakfast.'

What sort of questions to ask

Ask open-ended questions, not questions that require a yes or a no (these are what are known as closed questions). So, instead of asking, 'Do you feel sad about it?' (closed question requiring a yes/no answer) ask, 'What do you feel about it?' (open-ended question). A child wanting to please may say 'Yes' to a closed question – ('Yes, I do feel sad') just to agree.

For example, the child says, 'This is a story about a dog sitting in his kennel in the garden. All the people are in the house having tea. And so the dog is on his own.' The counsellor asks (wrongly): 'Was the dog feeling angry about that?' (This is a closed question that requires a yes or no answer.) Note that, here again, the counsellor imposes on the child her own thought of anger. The child has not mentioned anything to do with anger. In answering the question about anger, the child will have to move out of his particular feeling and imagining, and move into the thinking part of his brain to consider anger. (It transpired, in fact, that the dog was delighted to be in the garden, because all the people in the house were busy quarrelling, and the dog hated the noise!)

The counsellor should have said, 'I was wondering what the dog was feeling about being on his own when his family were having tea together?' (open-ended question).

Avoid 'Why?' questions. 'Why?' again means that a child must move away from his feeling and imagining to the thinking and assessing part of his brain. And he may not know why. Sometimes it just is!

The following are good interviewing questions for a central emotionally charged figure or object in a child's story:

- What is life like for him?
- Where does he live?
- What does he like to do most in the world?
- What does he like to do least in the world?
- What frightens him?
- What pleases him?
- What is the best thing about his life?

- What is the worst thing about his life?
- What or who does he love?
- What or who does he hate?
- What does he dream about doing with his life?
- What are his innermost secrets?

Useful questions if a child is enacting a story without words, or without obvious feeling content, include the following:

- What's happening now?
- What is X feeling about Y?', for example: 'What is the little tadpole feeling about being sat on by the two fat frogs?'
- What's going on now?
- What might X say if he could talk?', for example: 'What might the hedgehog say if he could talk?'

Such questions can also deepen the process of imagining. But avoid over-questioning and so turning the conversation into the Spanish inquisition! A child will often give you feedback if you do: by clamming up, losing interest in his story, or wanting to do something else instead. One little boy tried putting sellotape over his counsellor's too-eager mouth.

Things to do and say when working with a child's story

Encouraging the child in the rehearsal of the possible

Through story the child can rehearse a more potent and creative way of being in the world. Sometimes, however, children are on the verge of wanting to rehearse 'the possible' through their story, and yet, without encouragement, pull back from doing so. Often this is because of sabotaging voices in their head, or from a fear of being shamed or criticised. For example, one very depressed and oppressed child called Adam, who had been too good in class all year, started to come alive. One day he drew a picture of a magic helicopter. His teacher asked him about it. Adam told her a lovely story about how the helicopter flew into the highest clouds and made them twinkle with multi-coloured dust. At the end of telling his story, Adam said, 'I feel like getting in the helicopter and flying round the room.' If the teacher had not encouraged him in this rare surge of enthusiasm, this burst of life force, the moment would have been lost. With his teacher's encouragement, Adam flew in his imagined helicopter around the room, and all the children clapped. In that moment Adam tasted expansive life.

To similar moments of 'Shall I?', 'Dare I?', the listening adult can simply say, 'Do it' or 'Try it', or something encouraging like 'Sounds great, let's pretend this is your helicopter [large cushion] and this is the sky [space above child's head]', thereby setting up the conditions that will enable the child to imagine he is in a helicopter flying around the room. Use toys or any available props in the room to enact or rehearse the desired behaviour.

The mind can experience vividly imagined activity as the real thing, so 'rehearsal of the possible' in this way can be highly transformative. 'A good way to think of it is that energy follows thought. We need to be careful about what we imagine, for we may unknowingly become it' (Glouberman, 1989, p50). Consider the following examples:

Bobbie, aged six

For years, Bobbie had been an impotent victim to his much older cousin, who was constantly putting him down in very cruel ways. Bobbie had become very withdrawn and closed as a result.

Bobbie (after telling a story about a big, bad snapping-teethed mouth): 'I feel like sticking the bad mouth in a hole in the sand, and saying to it "No more!" so that it won't tell me I'm stupid any more.' He pauses. In this pause all this potent, taking-charge energy can die off if the listening adult does not respond.

Adult: 'Do it. Try it.'

Bobbie (does it, and grins from ear to ear): 'Yabadabadoo!!!'

Bobbie repeatedly rehearsed the possible like this in his stories over several weeks. Then, with the help of some adults in his life, he was able to confront his cousin and the bullying stopped.

Adult: 'So, Bobbie, how does it feel now you've stopped the bad mouth from saying horrid things to you?'

Bobbie: 'Like the best sort of day ever!'

This final exchange shows the importance of witnessing the child's potent action, and spending some time with it, so the child can strengthen and assimilate his feelings of potency.

The language of potency

For a withdrawn child who has been bullied, abused, oppressed or shamed, to then experience feeling potent and confident, active rather than passive, is a very important moment. It is far too important to leave unmarked. The child needs time to feel that moment physiologically as well as psychologically, and to process it so that it has an enduring positive effect.

Gitta, age seven

Gitta, who has been sexually abused, enacts a story about a little cat who gets yellow Playdoh all over her. Gitta says she finds it disgustingly grubby. The counsellor empathises with how awful the little cat must feel, being so smeared with yellow stuff which it has got right into its fur.

Gitta: 'Yes, yes, the cat feels "all spoilt".'

Gitta then starts to wash and wash the cat in the sink until it is very clean. She dries it lovingly.

Counsellor: 'What does the cat feel now that she's managed to get the yellow stuff out of her fur, and washed herself very clean?' Thus again the counsellor marks the moment of potency by asking Gitta what she feels about acting potently.

Gitta: 'Just lovely – clean and new, and now I'm building a wall with very big stop signs to stop the yellow Playdoh ever coming here again.'

Stories about being 'hopelessly stuck in a bog' (or its equivalent) may pose problems. Do you leave the child in the bog, or help him out of it? In answer to this, it is always a matter of whether the child needs you to really hear and understand how hopeless he is feeling, or whether he needs you to help him reconnect with some inner or outer resources he has in his life – ones which he has temporarily lost sight of.

Example A

The child tells a story about a lion stuck in the bog.

Counsellor: 'So how does the lion feel about being stuck in the bog?'

Child: 'Dreadful.'

Counsellor: 'How awful to have all that lion power and yet find yourself so powerless in the bog.' (empathy)

Child: 'Yes, it's just miserable. Like you say, the lion is used to feeling big, big, big – and now he's just a nothing.'

Counsellor: 'Is there anything he can do about it?' (language of potency/rehearsal of the possible)

Child: (answer 1): 'Well, he could call out to the little people in the tree at the other side to help him.'

Child: (answer 2): 'No, he feels he will just have to stay there until he dies.'

The 'language of potency' intervention – 'Is there anything the lion can do about it?' – is to be used with much caution. It may be that the child just needs his counsellor to stay with his painful feelings: in this case, despair and feelings of impotence and defeat. If the counsellor finds such feelings too threatening in herself, she may overuse the language of potency, and so push (consciously or unconsciously) the child to a happier, more hopeful place, when he is not feeling that at all! Rather, he may need her to really understand how defeated and hopeless he feels about something in his life.

Has the child, in answer 1, really retrieved some good inner resources with the support of his counsellor's question? Is he simply trying to please her? Or is he relieved that she has provided him with a nice neat means of escape from his more difficult feelings, such as how miserable and defeated he feels, like the lion in the bog?

Example B

Child (in his story): 'Oh no! The sheep has got a jellyfish on his head that's stinging it and stinging it. He just can't get it off, and he really wants to. It's driving him mad.'

Social worker: 'Is there anything the sheep could do to get the jellyfish off its head?' (a call for inner resources)

This social worker has come in too quickly here with the question about what can be done. She has not taken time to empathise with the sheep's pain and desperation at having this jellyfish on its head, stinging it and stinging it. It could be that the social worker is not able to stay with the child's pain about these attacks (which may well be a metaphor for painful emotional attacks in the child's life). The child may need the social worker to stay with his pain rather than trying to help him make it all better. For example:

Social worker: 'How awful for the sheep being stung again and again. He must be in a lot of pain, and I can really understand how he feels so desperate for it to end.'

Child: 'Yes he does, and no one is there to help him and he can't get the jellyfish off his head by himself.'

Social worker: 'And I'm thinking how terribly lonely for the sheep, and that his aloneness may feel at times as painful as the pain of the stinging jellyfish. How very, very sad that no kind sheep or person comes to help.'

Here the social worker has not moved straight into 'What could the sheep do?', so she has not blocked the child's important communication of feeling all alone and helpless and utterly unsupported in his pain. She may now stay with his pain. Alternatively, if it feels that the child is *also* moving into feeling anger and protesting, she may move into a question about resources: 'Is there anything the sheep can do?' If the child says 'No', it is again an important sign to stay more with the hopelessness, coupled this time with impotent anger.

Watching out for your presence in the story

Pete, aged 13

Pete has been psychologically abused by several mother-figures in his life, which has led him to have a deep mistrust of women. Pete is very tense. He knows no inner peace.

Pete: 'This story is all about a witch who turns the little boy into something else for a day and then forgets to turn him back.'

Therapist: 'What a very unsafe world the boy lives in, with people like that in it. I can imagine it would be very difficult for him to trust anyone or ever really feel he could let down his guard and just enjoy being in the world.' (empathy)

Pete: 'Too right!'

Therapist: 'And I'm just wondering if you feel that I might do that?'

Pete: 'Yes, I do. You might get inside my head, if I tell you anything about my life.'

Therapist: So I imagine it must be very unnerving for you being with me now.

Through the therapist's empathy and her acknowledgement of the child's transference on to her of his past experience of women, Pete could start to process his deep mistrust.

What to do if it is not clear who is who in a child's story

Some children's stories are very clear in terms of who is who: who are the bad guys and who are the good guys, and which characters represent the child and which represent other people in his life. Other stories can appear very confusing. You cannot just assume that, because there is a little baby and a big monster in a child's story, the child is identifying with the little baby. Lots of children, for example, have nightmares of monsters following a day in which they have had temper tantrums, because in a state of rage they can feel like a monster. It is also very common for children with depressed or exhausted mothers to tell a story in which the little hen, little duck, little cow and so on is their mother and they are the bad monster.

Figure 9 is an example of a 'who's who' story. It was enacted by John, aged nine, who at the age of six had a very frightening, cruel teacher. John had dreaded going to school ever since. John's story is about a man being attacked by monsters while lying on a grave.

So who is who? Is John telling what he would like to do to his frightening teacher, or is he telling what it felt like his frightening teacher did to him? It could be either, or both. Freud talked about 'condensation', meaning that, in dreams, one person can be 'a plurality of people', and one place can be 'a plurality of places'. So this story may be a 'condensed' image of John's feelings about the cruelty he experienced and his expression of rage at that cruelty. There are various ways of establishing the facts. First, you can use some of the interventions and questions detailed previously. Or you can ask overtly, 'Is he good or bad?' or 'Do you think he deserved such an attack?' Or you can use the 'nosy seagull' technique. This is a technique originated by Sue Fish, Co-Director of the Diploma in Child Therapy at the Institute for Arts in Therapy and Education, London.

After the child has told his story, nosey seagulls fly down. They settle down by the side of the child's enacted story and have a conversation. Often the child is so entranced by this unexpected piece of theatre enacted by the adult listener (via puppets or toys) that he tells the seagulls who is who in his story, and who is good and who is bad, and so on.

Dolly Seagull: 'Well, what do you think, Ethel Seagull? Was that big fat giant in the story good or bad? – because it did seem to be helping the little boy . . .'
Ethel Seagull: 'But Dolly Seagull, didn't you see it had enormous teeth. I never trust giants myself.'

Often the child can't resist.

Child: 'Look, sillies! Of course the giant is a good giant!'

The golden rule is: always hold firmly in your mind the *possibility* that a story character *may be a person in the child's life, or it may be an*

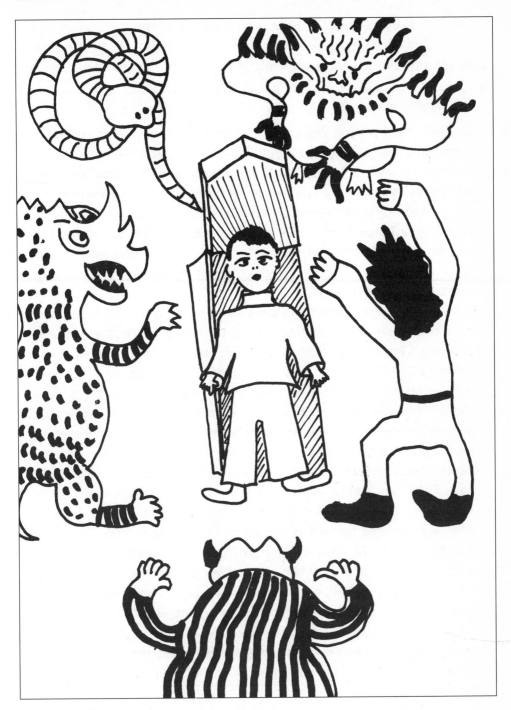

Figure 9 *Grave attack*

aspect of the child himself, or it may be both – a combined image. Never assume that a character is any one of these before getting clear information about it from the child. Consider the following example:

Izzy, aged seven

Izzy had spent several years watching his parents have terrible verbal fights, until they eventually split up. For several counselling sessions he enacted a story in the sandtray of one bloody war after another. In his stories, everyone in the war would be bombed and then they would die. In each of these sessions the counsellor had assumed (without checking up) that Izzy was identifying himself with the wounded. Indeed, Izzy had been psychologically very scarred by the trauma, and was very mistrustful with people, always expecting them to say something horrid to him.

Repeatedly, Izzy played the same story with no development, and so the counsellor realised she must be failing to read something properly. One day she decided to switch tack and said, 'Wow! What powerful bombers in the sky!' Izzy's face lit up – 'Yes, yes!', he said, dancing around the room. The counsellor had eventually got it right about who was who! Izzy had felt so desperately and unbearably impotent watching the war between his mother and his father that, in his imagination, via story, he needed to experience himself as potent, hence seeing himself as a powerful bomber. The counsellor then read him *A Wibble Called Bipley (and a few Honks)* (Sunderland & Armstrong, 2000), which is all about a little creature who felt so hurt and impotent that he turned to bullying to feel big and powerful and get away from his too painful feelings. This storytelling was to empathise more with Izzy about how people who have experienced terrible impotence often need to move into a feeling of power. Eventually, Izzy could communicate to his counsellor how he had felt so very helpless and frightened. After a while, he found a way to be powerfully creative as opposed to powerfully destructive, via his real success at computer studies and his story-writing in English at school.

'But I really empathised with the fear of the little bear in Polly's story, but Polly didn't say anything, so I thought maybe the little bear didn't represent her?'

Polly at age four is highly unlikely to respond directly to your empathy. Children are not like adults in counselling or therapy. Children do not say, 'Thanks, that's a really good intervention.' Often the only acknowledgement that your empathy is getting through will be that Polly's story or play moves on in some significant way. Also, at times after a truly empathic intervention, there is a tangible sense of relief in the room from the child's feeling deeply understood. The child might do something like climb on your lap and have a little sleep, or some other lovely relaxed just-being-together activity.

If you are empathising with the wrong character in the story, but for much of the time your capacity to understand has been good, it is likely that the child will repeat his story in some form or other until his message is received and understood. Then he will move on. And remember, sometimes stories are repeated, not because you have not understood something correctly – it is just that the child is working through and working through and working through. Digestion can be a long, slow process, particularly when something in the child's life has been very traumatic.

Working with the language of story with older children

Many older children (aged ten and above) are often more inhibited, and not so free initially with their imaginings. They tend to lose their capacity for spontaneous story-making and therefore need more support and structure from you, if they are going to journey into the realm of imagination for vital processing of their feelings.

With older children, if as a tool to inspire story you are using miniature toys and figures, you will often need to talk to them about this, otherwise they may well say 'Phooey, I'm not playing with toys. That's for kids.' You can explain that, although they may look like toys, they each stand for something. Then, placing something in the sandtray, you may say, for example: 'So someone might choose this shark to stand for their anger. Or they might choose this witch for someone in their life who is scary. Or they might choose this dead tree to stand for the times when they have felt bored or that everything was too dull.'

One tried and tested way to start a story session with an older child is to ask the child to make a picture in the sand, or to paint a picture. Say to the child that it can be a picture of something in his life, or just anything that comes into his mind. When he has painted his picture or done a picture in the sandtray, you could ask questions such as: 'Would you tell me about your picture?', or 'If it were a film set, what would happen next?' (If they have painted a picture, you can invite them to put miniature figures on the top of it if they like.)

They may then start to enact a scene or story, with or without words. So the still picture becomes a piece of drama in the theatre of the sandbox, or against the backdrop of the painting. The question, 'What would happen next?' has been a lifesaver for me on several occasions with some very troubled and inhibited older children and adolescents. For example, one girl would not talk to me for two years, but she would make pictures in the sandtray and she would show me what would happen next. It was rather like session after session of silent film. Eventually she told me verbally the story about her life, which she had enacted in metaphor for two years in the sand.

The technique of identification

After listening to the older child's description of their painting or sandplay picture without interrupting, you could ask: 'So, with all these images you have told me about, which are you most drawn to/which is the most powerful for you?' Once they have picked an image or set of images, you can consider interviewing them: 'So tell me, fed up sheep, what is life like for you in this world (of the sandpit, of the picture)?' 'What are you aware of/Not aware of?'

Ask the child to speak as 'I' (in the first person) when he is imagining himself into a particular story, object or image. This process is called *identification*. It can be a powerful technique which helps children really enter into their story with feeling, rather than just 'talking about' it. In other words, speaking as 'I' can bypass the censoring part of the brain and help transport the child firmly into the realm of imagination. If, for example, you are interviewing a cupcake which the child has put in the bottom of the sandtray, say, 'I'm asking you to be the cupcake, and I'll interview you to find out more about you.' Asking a child to identify with an image in this way can reach far deeper levels of clarity and truth.

The 'finish-the-sentence' interviewing technique

Using this technique, the counsellor says: 'So be the blue blob in your picture and finish the sentence, 'I am the blue blob and what I am feeling is . . .', or 'So be the drum-roll you have just played, and finish the sentence 'I am the drum-roll, and what I can do is . . .'.

Asking the child to 'finish the sentence' in this way provides him with a good support and he may feel far less embarrassed. Whereas if you just say, 'Be the prison bars in your story', or 'Be the squirrel', it can be most confusing for the older child. They may well say, 'But I'm not a squirrel!'

If a picture, story, sandplay and so on is crowded, it may be impossible (and unnecessary) to pay attention to all the images in this way in one session. If you only deal with one or two images in depth, and find the story hidden in those images, that is fine. For example, if the child is deeply involved with the relationship between a knitting needle and a cow pat in her sandtray picture, and does not refer to the other seven images in the sandtray, so be it. If the other symbols are important to the child they will recur in future sessions.

The technique of 'dialoguing'

'Dialoguing' is where two or more images in a child's picture or sandplay story clearly have an important relationship or connection (either conflictual or supportive), and you help them to converse. For example, in the sandtray a monster is standing on a small squirrel's head. This is clearly an important conflictual connection. Or, in a picture, a jagged red line is piercing a soft blue blob. In their stories, younger children will tend to enact a dialogue with two images or characters in powerful connection without any prompting, and give a natural running commentary about events, as in the following example:

Jake, aged six

'The big lorry comes and goes crash, crash into the little car.'

(Little car): 'Help help!'

(Tough big lorry speaking): 'I'm going to smack right into you, you deserve to get smashed up, you are too much of a wimp of a car.'

(Little car): 'You are right, I'm just a silly little wimp of a car.'

Jake had witnessed parental violence, and so was enacting here the feeling of an awful submission/dominance interaction he had seen.

Older children, however, will need supporting in the dialoguing of two or more important images that they have presented as being in relationship in some way. Asking them to engage in dialogue can reveal the story hidden in that picture or sandplay. The counsellor could ask: 'Would you be the squirrel, and talk to the monster?' or, offering a more holding structure, 'So, as the squirrel, could you finish the sentence, "What I feel about you, monster is . . .?"' Then she could get the child to switch, and ask him to be the monster and talk back to the squirrel and so on, back and forth in conversation. Be aware that these two characters may be the child and someone in his life, two people in his life, or two aspects of himself.

Identification and 'dialoguing' can be used with any theme or image provided by the child, for example:

Be your fear

Be the redness ('I am redness and what's very important about me is . . .')

Be the repetitive sound you played which you described as haunting.

Identification and dialoguing can also be used with any art form, such as music, play, poetry, puppetry, movement, drama, clay or art. *A word of caution*, however, about using dialoguing or identification as a technique: if a child is already feeling something very strongly and vividly with an image or story which he has created, using dialoguing and identification would be inappropriate and an interruption to the child. This is because dialoguing and identification are an aid to help the child go deeper into his imagination. If they are already there, they do not need this support.

How to end a session with a child who has told you his story

It is sometimes a good idea to do a summary of the story you have heard, and which you have worked through together. This is to show the child that you have really listened, and to help draw all the strands together, so the child can think more clearly about what he has just enacted. For example, you may say, 'So in your story today a big fish came and swallowed the world, and all the people were frightened and their houses got knocked down.' You may even say, 'I'm wondering if I've missed out anything important.'

Sometimes a child will also do something very important after working through his story with you, so provide the opportunity for this: 'Now we have talked all about your story, is there anything you would like to do or change in your drawing/sandpicture/play of your story?' Often, at this eleventh hour, the child will say 'Yes', and some miniature toy will get stamped on, thrown out, hugged, put on the adult's knee or shouted at. It is because something has shifted in the talking about, understanding and working through of the story. Again, whatever happens at this eleventh hour needs acknowledging by the listening adult.

Troubleshooting

'If a child does not move into a story – how can I help him to harness his imagination more deeply?'

Ask him if he would like to paint a picture or make something in clay or Playdoh. Then find the story hidden in the painting, or the clay or Playdoh model – there usually is one.

Child: 'Oh look, I've drawn a lollipop with a very sad face.'

Teacher: 'Hello, lollipop, nice to meet you. What is making you sad?'

In other words, interview the lollipop (see the 'good interviewing questions for a central emotionally charged figure or object in a child's story', listed on p65).

Child: 'Look at my painting – can you see how the red line is crashing into the blue blob, into everything in fact?'

Therapist: 'Oh yes, how does the blue blob feel about that? I'm wondering, what's making the red line want to do its crashing into things?'

or

Therapist: 'If it could talk, what would the blue blob say to the red line about being crashed into?'

Child: 'This is a clay tortoise.'

Therapist: 'Ah yes. Tell me about the tortoise . . .'

'What does it mean if the child keeps telling me the same story over and over, week after week?'

It usually means one or more of the following:

1 The child needs to tell this story a lot because he feels troubled, confused or disturbed by its emotional theme. He needs to keep trying to process his feelings about it via story. So the repetition of the story is a very important 'working through'.

2 The story includes some very important rehearsal of a different way of being, which again takes time. Children often need to rehearse a different way of being (for example, a softer, more gentler self, or a stronger, more assertive self) in fantasy via story, many times, before taking it into reality. Watch, however, for repeated rehearsal via story of self-destructive acts, which can occasionally happen. Although it is rare, children can rehearse such self-destructive acts as running away, self-harm or suicide attempts in story or painting, or through other creative media.

3 The child is stuck. He is trying to tell you something via story, and you are not hearing. So he has to keep telling you, hoping for that moment of real understanding, that moment of 'message received and understood'. It is the same with dreams, which can recur until their content is properly

felt and understood. They are then unlikely to recur, certainly not in that same form. If you are aware, you will sense when a child is stuck. There is a dull replaying of a story which comes from a kind of wearisome 'When are you going to get what I am trying to tell you?' You can ask the child directly, 'I wonder if I am not hearing something important in your story so that you are needing to tell it again and again?'

4   Sometimes, however, the child is stuck because he is telling his story through the wrong medium. For some children, for example, sandplay is too small for their very big feelings. They may need to tell you their story with percussion instruments, or by making some big stage set for it. Simon, aged seven, for example, got stuck in a repeated wearisome telling about people locked up in the tower of a fort. He told it through miniatures in sandplay. When the therapist suggested that they build a fort in the room using big cushions and a table, the story developed dramatically.

'What do I do if in his story a child is rushing on from one thing to another to another, flooding me (and probably himself) with images and feelings, so that nothing is being properly digested or worked through?'

Consider the following example:

Raja, aged eight

Raja tells the following story in the sandtray at immense speed:

'The bee turned into a monkey who was up in a tree, hanging by its tail. But it was scary because there were two bears below who wanted to eat him. Then the monkey–bee thing got pregnant. Then the monkey–bee thing fell against another tree, and the tree fell on top of the bears, and the bears were killed. And then along came a very frightened rabbit and had lots of babies, but a pig chased them. The monkey stepped on to the wings of the butterfly, so it couldn't fly away. Then the big beetle ate a sardine, but the sardine was still alive so it punched him from inside his belly and got out.'

Possible responses to this story which is so flooded with images and feelings:

Social worker: 'Phew, what a lot going on. If you were an animal in that world, what would you be feeling about all this going on around you?'

Social worker: 'What an amazing story. I really want to understand it, so I'd like to go back a bit to the beginning; I'm thinking of the first thing you said about the bee turning into a monkey and wondering about that, and what the bee felt about it.' (Then go through each of the images with time.)

Social worker: 'What an amazing story. Out of all those things that happened in your story, which are the most important things? (Getting the child to say where his main emotional charge is.)

If you are flooded with images like this, also take time if you can, during the session and afterwards, to really think about the main recurrent emotional themes in the story and the type of inner world and psychological landscape being presented. Instead of getting hooked on detail, think what you would feel like if you lived in a world such as that presented in Raja's story. It is a very unsafe, unpredictable, confusing and brutal world, with many threats to one's very survival and some actual deaths. There is a lot of unthinking cruelty, and a total absence of concern, kindness, shelter, safety, human warmth and so on (see, earlier in this chapter, the list of features to look out for in the psychological landscape in a child's story (pp50–53)). Raja also mentioned fear twice. Keeping within the metaphor, all this can be commented on and empathised with. There are some bits that you may never understand about this story, but that does not matter. What matters is that you empathise with the central emotional themes the child is trying to convey to you. (In reality, Raja did indeed live in a very unsafe world. Her father had died from a drug overdose, and her mother was an alcoholic.)

'What do I do with the problem of a child's inconclusive or half-expressed statements?'

Here are some suggestions:

Toby, aged seven, had a depressed mother. When she wouldn't play with him, he got very frustrated and sometimes hit her.

Toby: 'This is a story about a bulldozer sitting next to a rickety falling-down house . . .' (Being the bulldozer talking to the house): 'I want to smash you!'

Counsellor: 'I want to smash you because . . .?'

Toby: 'Because you are so weak and I am so big and tough!'

Counsellor: 'And when you are weak and I am so big and tough that makes me feel . . .?'

Toby: 'Very, very sad and very, very cross.'

Counsellor: 'So if the bulldozer could have a wish from the house what would it be?'

Toby: 'The bulldozer would wish from the house, "Be big and strong like me, then you could stop me trying to smash you up all the time".'

Counsellor: 'And I can understand how much the bulldozer wants that from the house. Because I guess the bulldozer really cares for the house, and so needs the house to help him to stop smashing it up.'

Toby: 'Yes, yes – the bulldozer thinks he is very, very bad because he hurts the house so much.'

Here the child spoke about some very important feelings. But he needed the counsellor to help him explore and speak more fully about his thinking and his feeling.

Incidentally, the counsellor did several parent-and-child sessions after this. She helped the mother to contain her little boy, so that they could have their relationship without this terrible war. The little boy was immensely relieved. He stopped hurting his mother. He threw his arms around the counsellor's neck and said, 'I love you'. Deep gratitude often engenders loving feelings.

'What do I do when a child inhibits himself in his play?'

The following are ways of handling this problem.

Child: 'I mustn't make a mess.'

Therapist: 'What are you saying to yourself in your head that means you can't make a mess now?'

Child: 'I shouldn't do it.'

Therapist: 'Can you find some puppets to be those voices in your head, and talk as them? What do they say, and how do they say it?'

Or

Therapist: 'Now what do you want to say to your shoulds? Find a puppet to be you, and talk to the should voices in your head.'

'But he's a very defensive child. Will he really speak to me through story?'

For inhibited, frightened or withdrawn children, you might like to help them get started by doing the 'telling a story together game'. Here is how it works. You have a big piece of paper between you and some crayons, and then you take it in turns to tell a bit of the story. You both draw what you are speaking about. But you start off the story making sure you include some reference (via indirect expression of course) to the troubling emotional issue with which the child is grappling. Here is an example:

Counsellor: 'OK, I am going to start a story. Once upon a time, there was a teeny weeny chipmunk in a too-big world, and every time someone shouted, he got smaller and smaller [being bullied and feeling shamed and powerless is the highly-charged emotional theme for this particular child]. And one day he was walking to the chip shop when . . . – You do the next bit.' (Passes crayon to the child.)

Child: 'Along came a horrid bully and smacked him in the face. And he just fell to the ground and sat there.' (Passes crayon to therapist.)

Counsellor: 'And he felt just awful and terribly, terribly alone [empathy], and then what happened was . . .'

Child: 'He saw a funfair in the distance.'

And so on.

After you have brought in the troubling emotional issue within some metaphorical context, make sure you keep empathising with the child's content. Do not take the story in the direction you want it to go, or bring in other emotional issues or your own feelings, which would just clutter the central theme. Any interventions you make about actions or events need to be neutral: they are simply there to help the child speak.

By and large, however, whether or not a defensive child will eventually speak through story to a parent, counsellor, teacher or social worker, usually depends on whether he feels his message will be heard. If he does not, he may just want to play ball or its equivalent instead, something which makes no journey into the realm of his imagination. Children are acutely aware of the capacity of a listener to understand and psychologically hold them through their most troubled feelings, their deepest pain. So if one child after another is not wanting to journey into the realm of the imagination with you, or starts but then gives up, ask yourself, 'Do I really know and dare to feel my own most troubled feelings and deepest pain?'

'When can I come out of his story world and the metaphor and talk about his real life?'

If the child talks about his real life to you – fine. He is letting you in. At other times, step with much caution out of the metaphorical and into the real. Remember that, by and large, children choose metaphor and story as their natural language for feeling, and do so because its indirect expression offers them protection. Also it is good to remember that all the healing work can happen entirely through your empathising *within the metaphor of the story*, so talking about real life is certainly not necessary for resolution and change.

If you do, however, venture into real life, do it tentatively and in a way that does not require an answer if the child does not want to give you one. But if you get a 'keep out' response or a resounding silence, respect it. You may say, 'I'm wondering if you ever feel like the squashed worm in your picture?', or 'I'm thinking whether you ever feel like the volcano in your drawing?', but let these be gentle wonderings 'into the air', so that, if the child wants to ignore them, he can.

If, however, a child has already ventured personal information about himself or his family, it gives you more licence to muse on connections, but again with caution and respect. For example, 'I'm thinking, the little boat swept over by the too big waves in your story today, reminds me of what you said last week about sometimes feeling you are drowning in your Mummy's sadness.'

Debs, aged seven

Debs had told her residential social worker all about her family being noisy and messy, with too many people in the house, and she wished sometimes that she lived on the moon because there were no people on it. Then one day Debs told a story about a little frightened worm who lived in an upside-down world with an upside-down sky, where everything fell out of everything because it was all so upside down.

Social worker: 'I'm thinking about your story and it reminds me about what you said about your family being too confusing, with too much noise and mess – and I'm wondering if that feels unsafe and frightening for you at times, just like for the worm in your story.'

Also, with an older child who regularly comes out of metaphor and talks about actual life events with you, you have far more licence to make references to real life. So you might say:

- 'Your stories keep showing things crashing into things. Does that ring bells for you in your life? I'm wondering if you ever feel that some people in your life are crashing into you like that in some way.'
- 'I am wondering if there is anyone in your life who you would like to crash into like that?'
- 'So in this story and in last week's story, a character is left all alone, with no one to help. Does that feel like something you know about or have known about in your life?'

But this 'licence' is not always available. Some older children and adolescents will still want the protection of the metaphor. In some sessions, they will want to stay in the metaphor, and they will want you to stay there too; in other sessions, they will want to tell you about real life, and so they are happy for you to talk about it too.

At the end of the session you might also ask something like, 'Is there any new or clearer thinking or feeling you are taking away from this session?'

All that now remains is for me to wish you well on your journeys into the realm of story. And if your co-traveller is a child who is open to the riches of this realm, the journey will indeed contain many treasures.

Bibliography

Armstrong-Perlman E, 1991, 'The Allure of the Bad Object', *Free Associations* 2(3)23, pp343–56.

Armstrong-Perlman E, 1997, personal communication.

Bettelheim B, 1975, *The Uses of Enchantment*, Knopf, New York.

Bollas C, 1987, *The Shadow of the Object: Psychoanalysis of the Unthought Known*, Free Association Books, London.

Brown J, 1996, *In A Woman's Likeness*, Todmorden, Arc.

Cardinal M, 1993, *The Words to Say It: An Autobiographical Novel* (trans P Goodheart), Women's Press, London (originally published in French, 1975).

Collingwood RG, 1958, *The Principles of Art*, Oxford University Press, Oxford (originally published by The Clarendon Press, 1938).

Comte F, 1994, *The Wordsworth Dictionary of Mythology* (trans A Goring) Wordsworth Editions, Ware (originally published in French, 1988).

Davis M & Wallbridge D, 1981, *Boundary and Space: An Introduction to the Work of DW Winnicott*, Karna/Brunner Mazel, London.

De Zulueta F, 1993, *From Pain to Violence: The Traumatic Roots of Destructiveness*, Whurr, London.

Dewey E, 1934, *Art as Experience*, Perigee Books, New York.

Ehrenzweig A, 1971, *The Hidden Order of Art: A Study in the Psychology of the Artistic Imagination*, University of California Press, Berkeley/Los Angeles.

Euripides, 1994, *Plays: One (Medea; The Phoenician Women; The Bacchae)*, Methuen, London.

Ferenczi S, 1930, 'Child-Analysis in the Analysis of Adults', pp126–42, in *Final Contributions to the Problems and Methods of Psychoanalysis*, 1995, Basic Books, New York.

Freud S, 1915, 'Repression', pp139–57, in *On Metapsychology: The Theory of Psychoanalysis*, Vol 11 of *The Penguin Freud Library* (Richards A and Strachey J, eds; Strachey J, Trans), 1991, Penguin, Harmondsworth, Middlesex.

Freud S, 1917, 'General Theory of the Neuroses', pp281–517 in *Introductory Lectures on Psychoanalysis*, Vol 1 of *The Penguin Freud Library* (Richards A and Strachey J, eds; Strachey J, trans), 1991, Penguin, Harmondsworth, Middlesex.

Gersie A & King N, 1990, *Storymaking in Education and Therapy*, Jessica Kingsley, London.

Giovacchini PL, 1989, *Countertransference Triumphs and Catastrophes*, Jason Aronson, Northvale, NJ.

Glouberman D, 1989, *Life Choices and Life Changes Through Imagework: The Art of Developing Personal Vision*, Unwin Hyman, London.

Greenberg JR and Mitchell SA, 1983, *Object Relations in Psychoanalytic Theory*, Harvard University Press, London/Cambridge.

Hillman J, *Interviews*, Spring Publications, Dallas, Texas.

Langer SK, 1953, *Feeling and Form: A Theory of Art Developed from 'Philosophy in a New Key'*, Routledge & Kegan Paul, London.

Lewis, CS, 1966, *A Grief Observed*, Faber & Faber, London (originally published 1961).

Lowenfeld M, 1991, *Play in Childhood*, MacKeith Press, London.

McNiff S, 1992, *Art as Medicine*, Piatkus, London.

Mills JC & Crowley RJ, 1986, *Therapeutic Metaphors for Children and the Child Within*, Brunner/Mazel, New York.

Moore T, 1992, *Care of the Soul: A Guide for Cultivating Depth and Sacredness in Everyday Life*, HarperCollins, New York.

Person ES, 1996, *The Force of Fantasy*, HarperCollins, London.

Polster E, 1987, *Every Person's Life is Worth a Novel*, WW Norton, New York.

Quiller-Couch A (ed), 1979, *The Oxford Book of English Verse 1250–1918*, Oxford University Press, Oxford.

Robbins A, 1986, *Unlimited Power: The New Science of Personal Achievement*, Simon & Schuster, New York.

Robertson J & Robertson J, 1969, 'John – 17 Months: Nine Days in a Residential Nursery', 16mm film/video, The Robertson Centre; accompanied by a printed 'Guide to the Film' series, British Medical Association/Concord Film Council.

Ross T, 1986, *I'm Coming to Get You*, Puffin, Harmondsworth.

Rowan J, 1986, *Ordinary Ecstasy: Humanistic Psychology in Action*, Routledge & Kegan Paul, London.

Rowsham A, 1997, *Telling Tales*, Oneworld, Oxford.

Share L, 1994, *If Someone Speaks, It Gets Lighter: Dreams and the Reconstruction of Infant Trauma*, Analytic Press, Hillsdale, NJ.

Storr A, 1972, *The Dynamics of Creation*, Penguin, Harmondsworth.

Sunderland M, 1993, *Draw on Your Emotions*, Speechmark, Bicester.

Sunderland M & Armstrong N, 2000, *A Nifflenoo Called Nevermind*, Speechmark, Bicester. (Storybook & Guidebook)

Sunderland M & Armstrong N, 2000, *A Pea Called Mildred*, Speechmark, Bicester. (Storybook & Guidebook)

Sunderland M & Armstrong N, 2000, *A Wibble Called Bipley (and a few Honks)*, Speechmark, Bicester. (Storybook & Guidebook)

Sunderland M & Armstrong N, 2000, *The Frog who Longed for the Moon to Smile*, Speechmark, Bicester. (Storybook & Guidebook)

Sunderland M & Armstrong N, 2000, *Willy and the Wobbly House*, Speechmark, Bicester. (Storybook & Guidebook)

Van der Kolk BA, 1989, 'The Compulsion to Repeat the Trauma: Re-enactment, Revictimisation and Masochism', *Psychiatric Clinics of North America*, 12: pp389–411.

Van der Kolk BA, McFarlene ACK, Weisaeth L (eds), 1996, *Traumatic Stress – the Effects of Overwhelming Experience on Mind, Body and Society*, Guildford Press, New York.

Wickes FG, 1988, *The Inner World of Childhood: A Study in Analytical Psychology*, 3rd edn, Sigo Press, Boston, MA.

Winterson J, 1995, *Art Objects*, Jonathan Cape, London.

Zinker J, 1978, *Creative Process in Gestalt Therapy*, Vintage, New York.

Index

Page numbers in italic indicate illustrations

Helping Children With Feelings

Margot Sunderland, illustrated by Nicky Armstrong

The titles in this extraordinary series are a vital resource for anyone working in child mental health. The practical guidebooks, each with an accompanying beautifully illustrated storybook, have been written to help children (aged 4–12 years) think about and connect with their feelings.

The guides and stories enable therapy professionals and teachers to work with a child to resolve a particular issue that may be worrying them, whether it's being a bully, rage, the loss of a loved one, anxiety or low self-esteem. They are also an extremely effective communication tool for parents to use with their children.

Each guidebook focuses on a key feeling and is written in very user-friendly language, covering the most relevant psychotherapeutic and neurobiological theories for that feeling.

Each guidebook:

- Includes what children themselves have said about what it is like for them; how they have coped with the feeling in ways which cause harm to self or others, and the consequences of that, and how they could have coped well.

- Provides exercises, tasks and ideas for things to say and do to help children. The exercises and ideas are specifically designed to help a child think about, express and process the feeling to the point of resolution. Many of the exercises offered will support children in finding creative, imaginative and playful ways to communicate their feelings.

- Enables child professionals to recognise the unresolved feeling behind the behaviour and to respond correctly to help the child work through that feeling to the point of resolution.

Guidebooks in the *Helping Children with Feelings* series include:

Helping Children with Fear

Helping Children Locked in Rage or Hate

Helping Children with Low Self-Esteem

Helping Children with Loss

Helping Children who are Anxious or Obsessional

Helping Children who Yearn for Someone They Love

Helping Children Pursue Their Hopes and Dreams

Helping Children who Bottle Up Their Feelings

*Helping Children who have Hardened
    Their Hearts or Become Bullies*

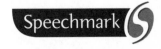